THE COMPLETE
Fibromyalgia
Health, Diet Guide
& Cookbook

—— Includes ——
Practical Wellness Solutions
& **100** Delicious Recipes

Dr. Louise S. McCrindle
B.Sc. (Hons), ND
& Dr. Alison C. Bested
MD, FRCPC

Robert
ROSE

For complete cataloguing information, see page 279.

Disclaimer
This book is a general guide only and should never be a substitute for the skill, knowledge, and
experience of a qualified medical professional dealing with the facts, circumstances, and symptoms of
a particular case.

The nutritional, medical, and health information presented in this book is based on the research,
training, and professional experience of the authors, and is true and complete to the best of their
knowledge. However, this book is intended only as an informative guide for those wishing to know
more about health, nutrition, and medicine; it is not intended to replace or countermand the advice
given by the reader's personal physician. Because each person and situation is unique, the authors
and the publisher urge the reader to check with a qualified health-care professional before using any
procedure where there is a question as to its appropriateness. A physician should be consulted before
beginning any exercise program. The authors and the publisher are not responsible for any adverse
effects or consequences resulting from the use of the information in this book. It is the responsibility
of the reader to consult a physician or other qualified health-care professional regarding his or her
personal care.

This book contains references to products that may not be available everywhere. The intent of
the information provided is to be helpful; however, there is no guarantee of results associated with
the information provided. Use of brand names is for educational purposes only and does not imply
endorsement.

The recipes in this book have been carefully tested by our kitchen and our tasters. To the best of our
knowledge, they are safe and nutritious for ordinary use and users. For those people with food or other
allergies, or who have special food requirements or health issues, please read the suggested contents
of each recipe carefully and determine whether or not they may create a problem for you. All recipes
are used at the risk of the consumer. We cannot be responsible for any hazards, loss, or damage that
may occur as a result of any recipe use. For those with special needs, allergies, requirements, or health
problems, in the event of any doubt, please contact your medical adviser prior to the use of any recipe.

Design and Production: Kevin Cockburn/PageWave Graphics Inc.
Editors: Bob Hilderley, Senior Editor, Health; and Sue Sumeraj, Recipes
Copy editor: Kelly Jones
Proofreader: Sheila Wawanash
Indexer: Gillian Watts
Illustrations: Kveta/Three in a Box
Eastern medicine illustrations: Louise S. McCrindle and Alison C. Bested

We acknowledge the financial support of the Government of Canada through the Book Publishing
Industry Development Program (BPIDP) for our publishing activities.

Published by Robert Rose Inc.
120 Eglinton Avenue East, Suite 800, Toronto, Ontario, Canada M4P 1E2
Tel: (416) 322-6552 Fax: (416) 322-6936
www.robertrose.ca

Printed and bound in Canada.

1 2 3 4 5 6 7 8 9 MI 21 20 19 18 17 16 15 14 13

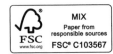

Contents

I dedicate this book to my husband, Randy —
for your reliability, support, strength and love over the past 35 years.
We've shared a wonderful life.
— Alison

I dedicate this book to my amazing husband, Craig,
and our beautiful twins, Evan and Abigail —
thanks for filling my life with so much love and beauty.
I love you.
— Louise

Acknowledgments

I would like to thank my co-author, Louise McCrindle, for inspiring the writing of this book. You are such an enthusiastic, caring individual who brightens the room when you enter it. How fortunate we have become friends.

I would like to thank my colleague, friend, and mentor, Dr. Lynn Marshall, who works at the Environmental Health Clinic at Women's College Hospital in Toronto, Ontario, Canada. She has been a wonderful teacher, source of inspiration, and support throughout our long struggle to teach doctors and patients about environmental medicine. I also want to thank the doctors at the Environmental Health Clinic, Drs. Riina Bray, Kathleen Kerr and John Molot, for our ongoing team effort on behalf of these patients.

I would like to thank the wonderful administration and staff at BC Women's Hospital and Health Centre and the government of British Columbia for helping me make my dreams come true by creating the Complex Chronic Diseases Program that helps patients with fibromyalgia, myalgic encephalomyelitis/chronic fatigue syndrome and Lyme disease. Together we will help make our patients' lives better.

Thank you to my patients for allowing me to accompany you on your journeys throughout the years. Your resilience, strength, patience, and hope continue to inspire me to fight on — on your behalf. Together we have laughed and cried and been encouraged in the process. I hope this book will help you if you suffer from fibromyalgia. I hope that it helps you to cope with your ongoing struggles and gives you coping strategies to improve your health.

— *All the best, Alison*

I would like to thank my co-author, Alison Bested, without whom this book would not exist. Thank you for being an amazing mentor, an inspiring and brilliant doctor, and a wonderful friend. I feel very privileged to have you in my life and I continue to learn and be inspired by you every day. Thank you so much.

Thank you to the Canadian College of Naturopathic Medicine for establishing the FM/CFS clinic. To all the faculty and staff and my incredible group of interns, whose enthusiasm and passion to learn and help others is infectious. Thank you so much.

To my outstanding colleague Sharon Kelly, who first introduced me to Alison Bested and who continues to be both a wonderful friend and mentor.

Thank you to my incredibly supportive parents, who have always encouraged me to follow my dreams and be true to self, which led me to this profession and continues to inspire my growth.

And last, but not least, thank you to my incredible patients, from whom I continue to learn so much and who inspire me to never stop learning.

— *Louise*

Introduction

Do you remember when you were normal? Your brain thought clearly and created balanced emotions. You usually felt that you had lots of energy for work or play, especially after a good night's sleep. You went about your day-to-day activities without excruciating pain. Now your brain is in a fog, you can't work due to the pain all over your body, you often feel exhausted and overwhelmed, your sleep is not refreshing, and you get anxious or depressed. Despite these problems, you push yourself to go on anyway.

Given these symptoms, you likely have fibromyalgia (FM), a medical syndrome that has been recognized only recently as a distinctive disorder with specific symptoms that can be treated. If you do in fact have fibromyalgia, you are not alone. According to the 2010 Canadian Community Health Survey, you are one of 438,900 people in Canada who have fibromyalgia. In the United States, you are one of an estimated 5 million adults.

Not so very long ago, fibromyalgia was thought to be a psychosomatic illness — it was all in your head — and received little attention from medical scientists and practitioners. There were few evidence-based studies being conducted in medical centers, and even fewer physicians were sympathetic to their patients complaining of these symptoms. Attitudes have changed, although there are some holdouts. It is still difficult to get a doctor to diagnose and treat you. Likewise, there are few books on fibromyalgia that provide a program for recovery and a cache of anti-fibromyalgia foods and recipes, as we do in this book.

The downward spiral of symptoms that characterizes fibromyalgia can be stopped. We now know that FM is caused by a combination of genetic and environmental factors that can be managed, if not cured, by a holistic application of medications, herbal medicines, exercises, and diet. We are convinced that a holistic approach is the only way to manage this complex medical illness.

In this book, we aim to help you understand fibromyalgia. What are the symptoms? What causes FM? Who suffers from this debilitating condition? We also present a plan for managing FM. Because we can't possibly treat everyone in our clinics, we have written this book to give you some common-sense tools that will help you to help yourself on your road to improvement and perhaps recovery. We use the SEEDS of health approach developed by Dr. Lynn Marshall at the Environmental Health Clinic at Women's College Hospital in Toronto, Ontario. Have patients recovered? Yes. And they stay recovered by continuing their efforts to balance and manage their lives. Do all patients recover?

Unfortunately, no; but most do improve the quality of their lives and learn to cope better with fibromyalgia.

We bring a unique set of knowledge and skills to bear upon this syndrome. Dr. Alison Bested is a hematological pathologist by training, and she has devoted the last 20 years of her practice to treating patients with fibromyalgia, myalgic encephalomyelitis/chronic fatigue syndrome, and multiple chemical sensitivities in her clinic and at the Environmental Health Clinic. More recently, she has been appointed the Medical Director of the Complex Chronic Diseases Program at BC Women's Hospital and Health Centre in Vancouver, British Columbia.

Dr. Bested has been fortunate to work with Dr. Louise McCrindle, a naturopathic doctor, for several years, helping patients with fibromyalgia. Dr. McCrindle is currently in charge of the Fibromyalgia and Myalgic Encephalomyelitis/Chronic Fatigue Syndrome Clinic at the Robert Schad Naturopathic Clinic, affiliated with the Canadian College of Naturopathic Medicine in Toronto. She also practices at the Bayview Natural Health Clinic in Toronto.

Our goal is to help you improve your ability to function and your quality of life. Our treatment approach is centered around rebuilding you: helping to reduce your pain, control inflammation, improve sleep, restore cognitive function (reduce brain fog), and increase your energy levels.

We start with the basics: you are what you eat. Another way of saying this is: garbage in, garbage out. But seriously, you can improve your body if you give it the basics to rebuild itself — good, simple nutritious food. This is what makes this book exciting. We have chosen easy-to-make, nutritious recipes and created shopping lists that will make it easier to conserve your energy at the grocery store.

By eating healthy meals and avoiding inflammatory foods, our patients have reported to us that their pain scores went down by an average of 10%. If you have chronic pain, you know that this can be the difference between coping and being in agony for the rest of the day.

This book is also a source of support. We have even included a simple letter to give to friends and family to help them understand your condition.

Our challenge to you is to try these suggestions and see if they work for you. We hope that this book gives you the support and resources you need to guide you on your path to health. We wish you all the best on your road to recovery.

Dr. Louise S. McCrindle, B.Sc. (Hons), ND
Dr. Alison C. Bested, MD, FRCPC

Open Letter for Support to Family and Friends

Date:

Dear _____,

I am suffering from fibromyalgia, but I am committed to returning myself to a state of health with your help. My journey will involve changes in my routine to make rest, nutrition, and self-care priorities. My doctor's experience and research both support the finding that rest is one of the most important factors to improving health in patients with FM just like mine. I need a time to rest and sleep. Rest in this context means having one's feet up and eyes closed in an environment free of excessive noise and bright light. FM patients don't respond to exercise in the same way that a person without this illness does. In my case, too much activity (mental, emotional, or physical) can leave me feeling suddenly depleted and needing rest. This up and down energy and other symptoms are frustrating for me and most patients with FM. Pacing myself and avoiding overdoing it on any one day, in any one hour, and taking rest breaks throughout the day will be one of the most important components of my treatment plan. I need to go to bed at a regular time. I need to stop pushing myself, and stop going to bed "wired and tired." I also need support in eating better meals — getting rid of junk food and eating more vegetables, fruit, and protein throughout the day to rebuild myself. These are not times to push through, as I have done most of my life; these are times to rest. It can be difficult to comprehend my experiences and the changeability of my symptoms, but these are typical in patients with FM.

Thank you for taking the time and interest to read this.
Yours in health,

_____

PS. I have difficulty asking for help. I would really appreciate it if you could: (check off the ones that apply)
- ❑ Call me once a week to keep in touch.
- ❑ Visit me once a month and bring dinner/lunch/coffee.
- ❑ Help me to organize and pay my bills.
- ❑ Help me grocery shop/grocery shop for me.
- ❑ Clean my kitchen.
- ❑ Do the laundry.
- ❑ _____.
- ❑ _____.

Part 1

Understanding Fibromyalgia

CHAPTER 1

What Is Fibromyalgia?

Case Study

Rear-Ended by Fibromyalgia

Claire was 54 years old and working full time as a grade 7 teacher when she was rear-ended in a car accident. This was the third time she had been in a car accident. The next day, Claire had a headache and felt pain in her neck and shoulders. She went to see her family doctor, who prescribed anti-inflammatory medication and recommended massage therapy. Over the next few months, her pain worsened. She rated the pain at 6 to 8 on a scale of 10 (with 0 as no pain, and 10 as the worst pain). She was unable to sleep. She went to bed exhausted and she woke up exhausted the next morning. Her pain spread to the rest of her body. At work, she spoke with her principal about her situation. She finally had to leave work when she couldn't remember how to teach a lesson to her students — one that she had taught many times previously. She is now on medical leave, struggling to go out grocery shopping for 20 minutes.

How Do You Know If You Have Fibromyalgia?

Fibromyalgia is a physical illness that is characterized by chronic pain felt all over your body and that has lasted at least 3 months. "All over your body" means that the pain is above and below your waist on both sides of your body, right and left. Having pain all over your body distinguishes fibromyalgia pain from most localized or regional pain syndromes.

Fibromyalgia Symptoms

Fibromyalgia pain has several other defining symptoms that may differ from patient to patient. This condition can also affect physical stamina (fatigue), sleep, and thinking (cognition). As a result of having to deal with the consequences of this chronic illness, some patients can become anxious or depressed.

Increased Pain Sensitivity: Sometimes even the lightest touch feels like pain if you have fibromyalgia. This increased sensitivity to pain is called hyperalgesia. The pain can be sharp or dull, or have a burning sensation.

Range of Pain Severity: Pain ranges from mild to moderate to severe. The pain can be constant or intermittent.

Location of Pain: Pain may settle in the muscles and joints, but there is no redness or swelling of the joints, as there is in rheumatoid arthritis. Sometimes the muscles feel knotted or bumpy. Sometimes the muscles have fasciculations, or are twitchy, like a tic of your eyelid.

Effect of Weather: Pain is worse with weather changes — notably when storms are about to arrive. The pain is worse with cold and damp weather and often improves in the summer with hot, dry weather. When fibromyalgia patients from north temperate climates escape the cold winter weather and fly south to a Caribbean island for a winter vacation, their symptoms improve while they are in the hot weather.

Associated Painful Conditions: Fibromyalgia also presents with other pain-related problems, such as migraine headaches, morning stiffness, temporomandibular joint syndrome (TMJ), irritable bowel syndrome (IBS), urinary bladder symptoms, and increased menstrual pain.

Fatigue Worsens with Exertion: In addition to the pain symptoms, you may also have fatigue, which is worse after exertion. Fatigue is often present. The fatigue may be mild, moderate, or severe.

Sleep Disorders: Fibromyalgia also presents with sleep problems, such as non-restorative sleep and sleep fragmentation.

Problems Thinking: Fibromyalgia patients experience difficulty with thinking (cognitive dysfunction), including the following symptoms: brain fog, poor short-term memory, or slowed processing.

Mood Problems: Depression and anxiety are found in many people who have fibromyalgia. This can be a result of having to cope with being chronically ill and in pain for a long time. Going without a diagnosis for many years — not knowing what is wrong — adds to this burden.

A 2013 study in behavioral medicine studied implicit memory function (meaning the type of memory where previous experience helps in the performance of the task without conscious awareness of it) in FM patients. FM patients were found to have "markedly reduced task performance." Of note was that depression, anxiety, and medication had only a very minor impact on performance. Rather, pain severity was most closely associated with lower implicit memory function and performance. The study concluded that lower implicit memory function is NOT due to motivational deficits.

The Language of Fibromyalgia

Fibromyalgia was first recognized as a medical condition in the 19th century and was called muscular rheumatism. Sir William Gowers called the combination of pain, stiffness, and disturbed sleep "fibrositis." This condition is now officially referred to as fibromyalgia syndrome. Like many medical conditions, there are a number of specific technical terms and a range of abbreviations used by health-care professionals that may be alien to you. Here are some key terms and their definition in plain language.

Fibromyalgia (FM): The term "fibromyalgia" has a compound meaning. "Fibro" means fibrous tissue (tendons and ligaments), "myo" refers to muscle, and "algia" means pain.

Syndrome: FM is a syndrome, not a disease. A syndrome is a group of symptoms and signs that together are characteristic of a specific condition, and the cause of the condition is not known. (A disease is a medical condition with recognizable symptoms that has resulted from a known cause.)

Myalgic encephalomyelitis (ME): "My" refers to muscles, and "algia" means pain. "Encephalo" refers to the brain, "myel" refers to the spinal cord, and "itis" refers to inflammation. So all together the term means inflammation of the muscles, brain, and spinal cord.

Chronic fatigue syndrome (CFS): Chronic fatigue syndrome is the same as myalgic encephalomyelitis and is the preferred WHO (World Health Organization) diagnostic name for this condition.

Q *What is the difference between fibromyalgia and myalgic encephalomyelitis?*

A That is a question we often hear. These two conditions have a large overlap in symptoms. FMS and ME patients can both have problems with fatigue, poor sleep quality, memory or concentration problems, pain in their muscles, and difficulty regulating the internal balancing mechanisms of their body, such as maintaining their blood pressure and heart rate. However, these conditions are not identical. ME typically starts after an infection — usually a flu-like illness — from which the individual has never recovered. FMS most often begins after repeated physical trauma, such as several car accidents that resulted in a head and neck injury. In ME, the diagnostic focus and treatment strategies focus on the fatigue syndrome, but in FMS, the focus is on the pain that begins as a localized head and neck pain and over time spreads throughout the body until the entire body has pain.

Q *How does fibromyalgia get started?*

A The answer to this question may come as a surprise. The patients we see have very similar histories or stories about how their fibromyalgia started. They are mostly women (80%) who are usually between the ages of 35 and 55. They have a history of physical trauma, usually in the head and neck area. They often have a history of being in car accidents at an earlier age. After the car accidents, they had treatments, such as physiotherapy and chiropractic treatments, and they recovered fully and were able to go back to work in their full-time career. Often the car accident before the onset of fibromyalgia was a whiplash injury where the head was snapped forward. Sometimes there was loss of consciousness. Often pain and muscle spasm began in the next few days or later that week. Patients often tried treatments that had worked for them in the past, but the pain continued and in fact worsened, spreading all over the body from the top of the head to the bottom of the feet.

Prevalence

Fibromyalgia appears to be growing in prevalence, in part because more and more medical practitioners are accepting the condition as a bona fide syndrome. In the United States, the prevalence of fibromyalgia is about 2% of the population, affecting an estimated 5 million adults. Prevalence is much higher among women than among men (3.4% versus 0.5%). In 2010, an estimated 438,900 Canadians had been diagnosed with fibromyalgia — over 80% were female. More than half of the fibromyalgia cases were between the ages of 45 and 64. Roughly one-quarter were younger than 45 years old, and 20% were 65 years old or older.

National ME/FM Action Network

For years, the National ME/FM Action Network has being telling government health officials that:

- Fibromyalgia is a very disabling illness.
- The illness has a substantial impact on people's lives.
- There are significant gaps in health-care delivery.

In the 2005 and 2010 Canadian Community Health Survey statistics, government data confirm these statements.

Canadian Community Health Survey (CCHS)

The Canadian Community Health Survey was a major survey designed to identify and monitor health issues affecting Canadians age 12 and up. From 29 million citizens, a sample size of 60,000 was taken for the 2010 survey, and the survey showed that Canadians with fibromyalgia have a poorer quality of life than Canadians in general. Topics addressed included levels of activity, socioeconomic disadvantages, and access to health care. The following charts are based on the statistics from the 2005 CCHS.

Access to Health Care

Patients with fibromyalgia receive health care less promptly than Canadians in general.

Percentage of group reporting on access to health care	Canadians with fibromyalgia	Canadians in general
Unmet health-care needs over the past 12 months	26%	11%
Unmet home-care needs over the past 12 months (age 18 and older)	11%	2%

Socioeconomic Disadvantage

These studies revealed that a greater percentage of people with fibromyalgia live at a lower socioeconomical level as compared to Canadians in general.

Percentage of group reporting on socioeconomic disadvantage	Canadians with fibromyalgia	Canadians in general
Permanently unable to work (ages 15 to 74)	14%	2%
Annual personal income less than $15,000 (age 15 and older)	43%	29%
Food source insecure	11%	5%
Very weak sense of belonging to local community	13%	10%

Activity Limitation

These studies also revealed that people with fibromyalgia have limited levels of activity as compared to Canadians in general.

Percentage of group reporting a need for assistance with daily activities	Canadians with fibromyalgia	Canadians in general
Need help preparing meals	16%	3%
Need help getting to appointments and running errands	28%	5%
Need help doing housework	35%	5%
Need help with heavy household chores (such as spring cleaning or yard work)	57%	12%
Need help with personal care	7%	2%
Need help moving about inside the house	8%	1%

CHAPTER 2

What Causes Fibromyalgia?

Case Study

An Unhappy Inheritance

Diane was really concerned. She felt like she was turning into her mother. Diane was now in her mid-40s, and she remembered that her mother had been sick for many years when she was in her 40s. She remembers that she had had difficulty sleeping, increased fatigue, and pain that seemed to get worse for a while. She remembers her mother having problems going to family reunions because the day was just too long for her. Her mother went to a rheumatologist, who said it wasn't arthritis but called it fibrositis. Her mom never complained and was now retired at age 68, but Diane knew that some days, her mother had a really hard time getting out of bed because she was so stiff in the morning. Diane made an appointment with her family doctor because she was now experiencing pain all over her body, she had difficulty sleeping, she had morning stiffness, and she was getting more fatigued over time.

From a Western medical perspective, fibromyalgia can be explained as the result of a genetic predisposition triggered by a combination environmental factors, such as physical trauma, poor exercise and sleep habits, nutrient deficiency, poor eating habits and pollution. From an Eastern medical perspective, fibromyalgia can be explained as an imbalance of yin and yang in the body. We have found that describing fibromyalgia from an Eastern medicine perspective is beneficial in terms of understanding the factors that are present at the onset of fibromyalgia and how these factors impact the body. This model helps to explain not only what may cause fibromyalgia, but also what treatments are needed for recovery from fibromyalgia.

Genetic Predisposition

We do not know the exact cause of fibromyalgia, but we do know that it is found more commonly in some families than in others — just like we know that high blood pressure or heart attacks run in some families. This is called a genetic predisposition.

Genetic Research

In one study, the genetic make-up of 1,500 patients with chronic fatigue syndrome and fibromyalgia was compared to normal healthy control subjects. The results were genetically analyzed using single nucleotide polymorphism (SNP) technology developed to make a map of our human genes. The fibromyalgia and chronic fatigue syndrome patients were genetically distinguished from normal controls. Research shows an increased risk with first-degree relatives. If your mother has fibromyalgia, you as her daughter are more likely to have fibromyalgia. Other research has shown the genes that help modulate pain interpretation by the brain may also be involved.

Another research trial, published in the journal *Arthritis and Rheumatism*, studied the genetic component of FM by genotyping 116 families. The results not only suggest a strong genetic component to FM, but also reported a "genome-wide suggestive linkage of fibromyalgia to the chromosome 17p11.2-q11.2 region." In other words, they were able to identify susceptibility loci (or region on a chromosome where mutations affecting one or more genes is present) for FM patients. This opens the door for much-needed future research.

Fibromyalgia Facts

- Fibromyalgia is a physical illness, not psychosomatic, as functional magnetic resonance image (MRI) studies, sleep studies, immune studies, and genetic studies have proven.
- Fibromyalgia affects women and children. It is most common in middle-aged women. It runs in families.
- Fibromyalgia does not have a single identifiable cause, but some people have a genetic disposition to fibromyalgia that is triggered by environmental factors. The most common trigger is physical trauma.
- Fibromyalgia patients have a higher risk of death from suicide than other patients. Fibromyalgia has a direct impact on emotional health as you grieve the loss of your health and try to find peace and joy while being chronically ill.

- Fibromyalgia treatment tends to be holistic, ranging from genetic therapy to cognitive behavioral therapy, to match the many causal factors.

Triggers

Although physical trauma to the head and neck is the most common trigger for fibromyalgia, there are other factors that can cause a total body burden that can result in fibromyalgia symptoms.

Total Body Load

Lack of Support

You may have no support in your life. For example, you are divorced, have teenagers living at home, and are dealing with aging parents. You are part of the sandwich generation — squeezed at both ends.

Poor Environment

You may live in a house that became moldy when your roof leaked. You seem to have a runny nose and itchy eyes when you are at home. You feel better when you are outside and at work.

You have noticed that if you eat a lot of potatoes or potato chips, you don't feel well the next day and you are wondering if you are having troubles digesting them. You feel bloated and uncomfortable after eating them. This is new for you.

You now have repeat infections, either bronchitis or urinary tract infections. It seems like you just get rid of one and you fall ill again.

You have eaten a lot of tuna in the past, because it is a cheap source of protein. Now you are worried that you have too much mercury in your body as a result. You read recently that exposure to mercury can be from the consumption of large cold-water fish (tuna, swordfish, and shark are examples), and from mercury dental amalgams.

Exercise

You know you need to get out with the dog for a half-hour walk every day, but you are just too tired to do it daily.

Diet

You are a good cook but lately have been picking up fast food because you are just too tired to go grocery shopping and cook all on the same day.

Sleep

You are so tired you want to sleep all day and night. When you do go to bed, you lie awake at night or keep waking up throughout the night. You get up in the morning more tired than when you went to bed. You used to work shifts with no problem, but now you don't recover after changing shifts.

Yin and Yang Imbalance

From an Eastern medicine perspective, good health is the result of maintaining an equilibrium between two forces of energy in the body, known as yin and yang. One is not better or worse than the other — ideally they exist in a state of balanced equilibrium. This means that in a state of health, there is an equal but fluid balance between yin and yang. One cannot exist without the other.

Yang	Yin
Male	Female
Expanding	Nurturing
Energy	Matter
Acute	Chronic
Fast	Slow
Short wavelength, high amplitude	Long wavelength, low amplitude
Hot	Cool
Fight or flight (sympathetic nervous system)	Rest and digest (parasympathetic nervous system)
Work	Sleep
Dryness	Water

Balanced Yang and Yin

Yang has a short wavelength and high amplitude, whereas yin has a long wavelength and a low amplitude. This means that yang is relatively quick to increase or decrease — it is more acute in nature. Yin is much slower-moving and has likely been depleting slowly over the course of years. For this reason, yin is not something that can be restored quickly.

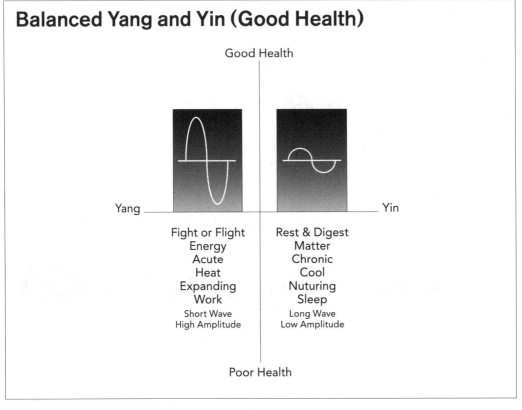

Balanced Yang and Yin (Good Health)

Good Health

Yang

Yin

Fight or Flight	Rest & Digest
Energy	Matter
Acute	Chronic
Heat	Cool
Expanding	Nuturing
Work	Sleep
Short Wave	Long Wave
High Amplitude	Low Amplitude

Poor Health

Eastern medicine illustrations courtesy of Louise S. McCrindle and Alison C. Bested.

Yin Depletion

We live in a society that tends to place a lot of value on the yang, particularly in the work environment. There is much value placed on drive, achievement, and accomplishment. Before becoming ill with fibromyalgia, you were likely very depleted of yin. Your health became unbalanced.

Factors depleting your yin:

- Overworking (drive)
- Poor diet
- Chronic stress
- Lack of sleep
- Trauma

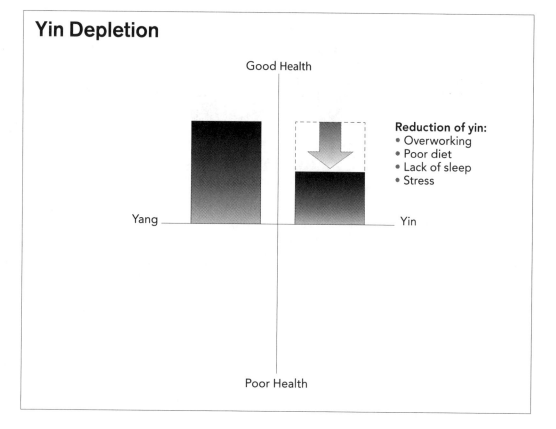

Running on Empty

In a "relative" sense, you found yourself with an excess of yang and you were low in yin relative to yang. You didn't have an excess of yang, but you simply had less yin to offset it. In other words, you were very depleted, running on false energy, or "running on empty." Some Eastern medicine practitioners would describe this as an adrenalin-like state or a state of "empty heat." You were living in a survival state of fight or flight, likely thriving off the false sense of energy and efficiency that can come with it.

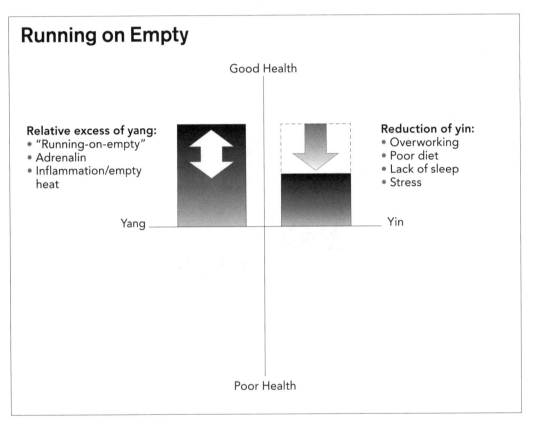

Running on Empty

Good Health

Relative excess of yang:
- "Running-on-empty"
- Adrenalin
- Inflammation/empty heat

Reduction of yin:
- Overworking
- Poor diet
- Lack of sleep
- Stress

Yang

Yin

Poor Health

Crash Cycle

Many people in Western society live their entire lives in this state of empty heat (or with relative excess of yang). When you are in this extremely depleted state, you may "crash," and fibromyalgia may be the result, especially if you have a genetic predisposition to fibromyalgia. Your first crash is likely the result of a physical trauma or repeated physical traumas. This trauma triggers a sharp decline in your yang, with no yin to balance and support it. You crash quickly, losing a lot of yang at once. In a "relative" sense, you have more yin than yang, but in fact you are now very depleted in both yang and yin.

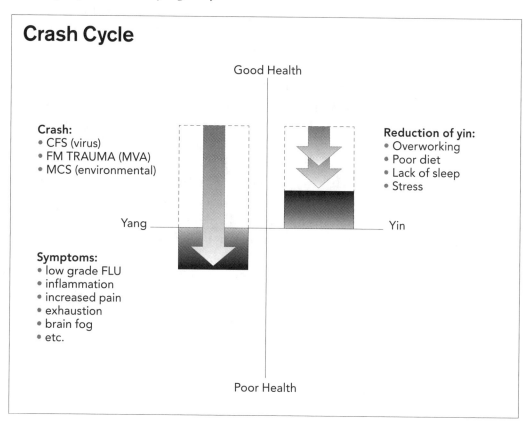

Crash Cycle

Good Health

Crash:
- CFS (virus)
- FM TRAUMA (MVA)
- MCS (environmental)

Reduction of yin:
- Overworking
- Poor diet
- Lack of sleep
- Stress

Yang _____ Yin

Symptoms:
- low grade FLU
- inflammation
- increased pain
- exhaustion
- brain fog
- etc.

Poor Health

Pain

If you look back to the definition of yin, this means that you have minimal energy (yang is now lower than yin), so you need to move slowly, you have a relative excess of dampness (yin is water), and this dampness is stagnant without the energy from yang to move it. In Eastern medicine, stagnation is pain. This also accounts for the worsening of symptoms in damp, cool weather and the sensation of brain fog.

Nervous System

From a nervous-system perspective, you are no longer in balance with your yin and yang energy and therefore have trouble regulating digestion, reducing inflammation, regulating immune function and sleep patterns, and controlling pain.

Crash Accumulation

From a yin-building perspective, each crash is more severe and reverses whatever progress has been made. Yang is relatively easy to rebuild because it is acute in nature and has a short wavelength and high amplitude. However, yin took years to deplete because it is chronic and slow-moving in nature. You can supplement or build back yang, but you will have nothing to stand on without yin. This explains the crash cycle as seen in fibromyalgia, and it helps us to understand why rebuilding yin is essential to recovery from fibromyalgia.

CHAPTER 3

How Is Fibromyalgia Diagnosed?

Case Study

Asleep on the Job

Helen is a 30-year-old woman who works as a professional accountant for a trucking firm. She has always worked long hours, and her employer has often commended her on her "drive." Lately, however, she has lost her drive. She has little energy left after work for her favorite activity, playing softball in the intercity league. She just wants to sleep, but sleeping is never refreshing. Her muscles have begun to ache, and at times, the pain is quite severe.

Helen went to see her family doctor because of her ongoing fatigue, difficulty sleeping, memory problems, and muscle pain. She was so tired that she was falling asleep at her desk in her accounting office. Her doctor examined her and found nothing out of the ordinary, so he ordered some blood tests to try to find out why she was so tired. The results of her blood tests were all normal.

By chance, her doctor had just returned from a medical convention and wondered if she had this new condition called fibromyalgia. He tested her fibromyalgia tender points, and she was positive for all 18 of them. He told her that she had this newly recognized condition.

Differential Diagnosis

There is no specific test for diagnosing suspected fibromyalgia. Rather, this condition is determined by differential diagnosis, ruling out associated conditions, and by matching symptoms to diagnostic criteria established by medical associations.

Standard Laboratory Tests

Basic laboratory testing should be conducted to rule out other causes of the symptoms of fibromyalgia. Here is a list of tests and the conditions they rule out.

Thyroid-stimulating hormone: to rule out an underactive thyroid or hypothyroidism (an endocrine disease that causes fatigue).

Complete blood count: to rule out anemias and blood conditions that can cause fatigue.

Liver function and kidney function: to rule out causes of fatigue.

Erythrocyte sedimentation rate, C-reactive protein, and creatine kinase: to rule out inflammatory diseases (such as multiple sclerosis), rheumatic conditions (such as arthritis and polymyalgia rheumatica), or neurological disease (such as myopathy).

Baseline testing of serum ferritin, serum B_{12} level, and serum vitamin D 25-hydroxy levels: to rule out iron deficiency or overload (serum ferritin), as well as vitamin B_{12} and D deficiencies; these deficiencies have an impact on the absorption of nutrients in the intestine and can affect energy levels.

Sleep study: to rule out causes of treatable sleep disorders, such as sleep apnea.

History of irritable bowel symptoms: to rule out inflammatory bowel diseases, such as Crohn's disease, ulcerative colitis, and celiac disease.

Food allergy diaries or allergy testing: to rule out sensitivities to foods if there are ongoing digestive problems.

Psychological testing: to diagnose reactive depression and/or anxiety in addition to fibromyalgia if you have symptoms of depression and/or anxiety.

Depending on a patient's clinical history, family history, and physical findings, appropriate additional testing may be required.

Questionnaires and Diagnostic Scales

Symptom questionnaires and pain scales are also helpful tools for assessing the impact of fibromyalgia due to the presence of pain, fatigue, and sleep problems. If new symptoms develop, they should be evaluated. It should not be assumed that they are part of fibromyalgia.

The American College of Rheumatology Preliminary Diagnostic Criteria for Fibromyalgia and Measurement of Symptom Severity 2010

This scoring system is used by doctors to help them to diagnose fibromyalgia in patients. The FM criteria are a combination of the Widespread Pain Index and the Symptom Severity Score.

Fibromyalgia Diagnostic Criteria

A patient satisfies diagnostic criteria for fibromyalgia if these 3 conditions are met:

❶ **Widespread pain index (WPI)** ≥ (greater than or equal to) 7 and **symptom severity (SS) scale** score ≥ (greater than or equal to) 5, or WPI 3–6 and SS scale score ≥ (greater than or equal to) 9.

❷ Symptoms have been present at a similar level for at least 3 months.

❸ The patient does not have a disorder that would otherwise explain the pain.

Part 1: Widespread Pain Index (WPI)

The WPI is a measure of the number of painful body regions that you have.

Determining Your Widespread Pain Index (WPI)

Check each area you have felt pain in over the last week. The final score will be between 0 and 19.

☐ Jaw — left	☐ Upper arm — left	☐ Upper leg — right
☐ Jaw — right	☐ Upper arm — right	☐ Lower leg — left
☐ Neck	☐ Lower arm — left	☐ Lower leg — right
☐ Upper back	☐ Lower arm — right	☐ Hip (buttock) — right
☐ Lower back	☐ Chest	☐ Hip (buttock) — left
☐ Shoulder girdle — left	☐ Abdomen	
☐ Shoulder girdle — right	☐ Upper leg — left	

Count up the number of areas checked and enter your Widespread Pain Index (WPI) Score here _____.

Part 2: Symptom Severity Score (SS)

The SS scale score is the sum of the severity of the 3 symptoms (fatigue, waking unrefreshed, cognitive symptoms) plus the extent (severity) of your other somatic/body symptoms in general.

Determining Your Symptom Severity Score SS (Score)

Check each area that applies to you in parts 2a and 2b. The final score is between 0 and 12.

Part 2a

Indicate your level of symptom severity over the past week using the following scale.

Fatigue

0 = No problem
1 = Slight or mild problems; generally mild or intermittent
2 = Moderate; considerable problems; often present and/or at a moderate level
3 = Severe: pervasive, continuous, life-disturbing problems

Waking unrefreshed

0 = No problem
1 = Slight or mild problems; generally mild or intermittent
2 = Moderate; considerable problems; often present and/or at a moderate level
3 = Severe: pervasive, continuous, life-disturbing problems

Cognitive symptoms

0 = No problem
1 = Slight or mild problems; generally mild or intermittent
2 = Moderate; considerable problems; often present and/or at a moderate level
3 = Severe: pervasive, continuous, life-disturbing problems

Tally your score for Part 2a (not the number of checkmarks) and enter it here _____.

Part 2b

Check each of the following OTHER SYMPTOMS you have experienced over the past week.

☐ Muscle pain
☐ Irritable bowel syndrome
☐ Fatigue/tiredness
☐ Thinking or remembering problems
☐ Muscle weakness
☐ Headache
☐ Pain/cramps in abdomen
☐ Numbness/tingling
☐ Dizziness
☐ Insomnia
☐ Depression
☐ Constipation

☐ Pain in upper abdomen
☐ Nausea
☐ Nervousness
☐ Chest pain
☐ Blurred vision
☐ Fever
☐ Diarrhea
☐ Dry mouth
☐ Itching
☐ Wheezing
☐ Raynauld's
☐ Hives/welts
☐ Ringing in ears
☐ Vomiting
☐ Heartburn

☐ Oral ulcers
☐ Loss/change in taste
☐ Seizures
☐ Dry eyes
☐ Shortness of breath
☐ Loss of appetite
☐ Rash
☐ Sun sensitivity
☐ Hearing difficulties
☐ Easy bruising
☐ Hair loss
☐ Frequent urination
☐ Painful urination
☐ Bladder spasms

Count up the number of symptoms checked on the previous page.* If you tallied:

0 symptoms   Give yourself a score of 0
1 to 10   Give yourself a score of 1
11 to 24   Give yourself a score of 2
25 or more   Give yourself a score of 3

Enter your score for Part 2b here _____.

Now add Part 2a AND 2b scores, and enter _____.
This is your Symptom Severity Score (SS score), which can range from 0 to 12.

What Your Scores Mean

A patient meets the diagnostic criteria for fibromyalgia if the following three conditions are met:

1a. The WPI score (Part 1) is greater than or equal to 7 AND the SS score
     (Part 2a & b) is greater than or equal to 5

OR

1b. The WPI score (Part 1) is from 3 to 6 AND the SS score (Part 2a & b) is greater
     than or equal to 9.
2.   Symptoms have been present at a similar level for at least 3 months.
3.   You do not have a disorder that would otherwise explain the pain.

For example:
• If your WPI (Part 1) was 9 and your SS score (Parts 2a & b) was 6, then you would
  meet the new FM diagnostic criteria.
• If your WPI (Part 1) was 5 and your SS score (Parts 2a & b) was 7, then you would
  NOT meet the new FM diagnostic criteria.

* The FM diagnostic criteria did not specify the number of "Other Symptoms" required to score the point rankings from 0 to 3. Therefore, we estimated the number of symptoms needed to meet the authors' descriptive categories of: 0 = No symptoms; 1 = Few symptoms; 2 = A moderate number; 3 = A great deal of symptoms.

This survey is not meant to substitute for a diagnosis by a medical professional. Patients should not diagnose themselves. Patients should always consult their medical professional for advice and treatment. This survey is intended to give you insight into research on the diagnostic criteria and measurement of symptom severity for fibromyalgia.

Adapted from Wolfe F, et al. The American College of Rheumatology preliminary diagnostic criteria for fibromyalgia and measurement of symptom severity. Arthritis Care Res. 2010;62(5):600–610.

For the purpose of epidemiologic and clinical research, the fibromyalgia criteria and severity scales were modified in 2011. Reference: Wolfe F, et al. Fibromyalgia criteria and severity scales for clinical and epidemiological studies: A modification of the ACR preliminary diagnostic criteria for fibromyalgia. J Rheum. 2011;38(6):1113–22.

Pain Rating Scales

Using visual analog scales, you can describe your pain level at its worst and its best. The higher the number, the worse the pain. At the far end, 10 means it is your worst pain — compared with 0, which means you have no pain. These scales are not only effective for diagnosing the degree of pain, but also for monitoring the effectiveness of pain treatments.

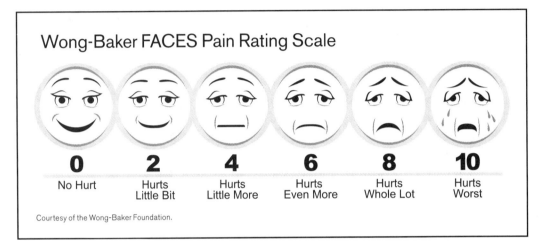

Wong-Baker FACES Pain Rating Scale

0	2	4	6	8	10
No Hurt	Hurts Little Bit	Hurts Little More	Hurts Even More	Hurts Whole Lot	Hurts Worst

Courtesy of the Wong-Baker Foundation.

18 points (9 front, 9 back) used to diagnose fibromyalgia

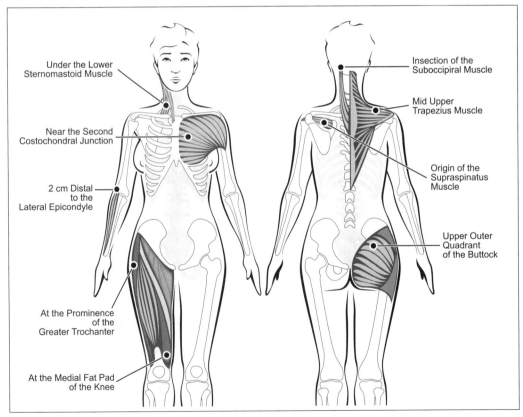

Under the Lower Sternomastoid Muscle

Near the Second Costochondral Junction

2 cm Distal to the Lateral Epicondyle

At the Prominence of the Greater Trochanter

At the Medial Fat Pad of the Knee

Insection of the Suboccipiral Muscle

Mid Upper Trapezius Muscle

Origin of the Supraspinatus Muscle

Upper Outer Quadrant of the Buttock

Adapted from the American College of Rheumatology, 2010.

Consensus Guidelines

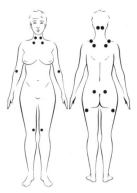

For many years, fibromyalgia was a homeless medical condition, recognized as a real disease by few medical practitioners outside of a small number of rheumatologists and environmental health professionals. Even when ignored, fibromyalgia would not go away and was eventually recognized by the American College of Rheumatology, which established a set of consensus standards and guidelines for fibromyalgia. These guidelines have evolved as we have been better able to understand this syndrome.

❶ In 1990, the American College of Rheumatology published the first guidelines for diagnosing fibromyalgia.

- History of widespread pain lasting for a minimum of 3 months
- Response from at least 11 out of 18 positive tender points, or specific locations on the body that are painful with the application of 8 pounds (4 kg) of pressure at that site

❷ In 2004, the original definition of fibromyalgia was updated and the condition was renamed fibromyalgia syndrome. Other diagnostic criteria were also added, including fatigue, sleep disorder, memory problems (brain fog), heat or cold intolerance, emotional numbness or anxiety, autonomic dysfunction (difficulties regulating blood pressure and heart rate), marked weight change, and morning stiffness.

❸ In 2010, the American College of Rheumatology eliminated the tender-point examination in favor of three questionnaires and indices.

- *Pain Scale:* The widespread pain index (WPI) is ≥ 7 and the symptom severity score (SS) is ≥ 5, or the WPI is 3 to 6 and the SS ≥ 9.
- *Duration:* Symptoms have been present at a similar level for at least 3 months.
- *Differential Diagnosis:* The patient does not have a disorder that would otherwise explain the pain.

This established the diagnosis of fibromyalgia without needing to use the tender-point physical examination. It has helped to diagnose men who had fibromyalgia but who were previously undiagnosed (men often do not have positive tender points). However, in 2010, most doctors did not have these questionnaires readily available in their offices, so overall, these questionnaires and indices were not very helpful.

❹ In 2012, the Canadian Guidelines for the Diagnosis and Management of Fibromyalgia Syndrome were released. Several guidelines and standards were established. Here are some of the highlights.

Early diagnosis

"An early diagnosis will allow attention to be focused toward symptom management, attainment of optimal health, and maintenance or improvement of function."

Primary care

"The responsibility for the diagnosis and management of FM should be shifted away from the specialist (rheumatologist) and concentrated in the primary-care setting. Specialist confirmation or fulfilling diagnostic criteria is not required."

Medical Training

Although early diagnosis and treatment is certainly a standard that all health-care professionals should abide by, the concept of asking family practitioners to take full responsibility for diagnosing fibromyalgia is not realistic at this time. Why? Because many family doctors have not been taught how to diagnose or treat patients with fibromyalgia. Fibromyalgia is a complex illness with many symptoms. In the past, it has been handled by rheumatology specialists because they were the ones who first identified fibromyalgia as a separate condition and have been trained to diagnose it.

Due to the recent introduction of several medications that have been helpful in managing fibromyalgia, this is beginning to change, but we are not at the tipping point yet.

Did You Know?

Confirming the Diagnosis

There are no specific tests that can confirm the diagnosis of fibromyalgia. The diagnosis is based on the history of widespread pain all over the body and includes other symptoms, such as unrefreshing sleep and poor memory and concentration. Having 11 out of 18 tender points is helpful, but this is not absolutely necessary to make the diagnosis, especially in men, who often do not have positive tender points.

Managing Fibromyalgia

CHAPTER 4
SEEDS of Health Program

Case Study

Start Low and Go Slow

Margaret is a 49-year-old woman with severe fibromyalgia who is struggling to find a way to manage her symptoms. She is on medical disability because her energy level is so low. On a scale of 10, she rates her energy level between 4 and 5. A normal energy level is 9 to 10 out of 10.

From time to time, Margaret has great days when her energy level is higher, about 6 out of 10. She usually walks about 10 minutes daily, but on these good days, she becomes more ambitious. A few days before she came to our clinic for a checkup, she decided to go shopping at the mall. She walked around for about an hour but became so tired she had trouble getting home on the bus. She crashed in bed for the next 2 days and lost any gains she had made in managing her fatigue and pain.

During her checkup, we took the time to review the concept of pacing with Margaret once again. It is a simple concept but difficult for many patients to get the hang of. We explained that she needed to pace herself while doing daily activities, such as shopping, and that overextending herself could spoil a good day. All of her efforts to improve went up in smoke when she crashed by overdoing the exercise — shopping for too long a time. We encouraged her to start again and to use her activity log to chart daily activities and related symptoms, and we scheduled another visit to work through this log to see how important pacing is for improving fibromyalgia. In Margaret's case, it meant that on a good day she could increase her walking by 10%, going from 10 minutes to 11 minutes in total walking time. A motto for patients recovering from fibromyalgia is "Start low and go slow."

How can fibromyalgia be treated? There is no single treatment that works for everyone, which means that you may need to combine elements of several therapies to find the mix that best suits your symptoms. Fibromyalgia affects many body systems and may require many different treatments to manage them. Although fibromyalgia cannot be "cured" with a magic bullet or a quick fix, many people with fibromyalgia are nevertheless able to improve their quality of life and, in some milder cases, experience recovery by adopting these therapies.

Management Principles

The traditional treatments for fibromyalgia are complex and overlapping. It is not as simple as prescribing a pill that will make it all go away. Our approach is holistic, personalized, patient-centered, and team-oriented.

Holistic

Holistic medicine has three areas of focus related to fibromyalgia care. First, holistic medicine focuses on the care of the whole person, treating the body, mind, and spirit as one. Second, holistic medicine integrates conventional and complementary therapies to promote optimal health. All appropriate healing modalities can be used — from medication to meditation, from homeopathy to herbal medicine — provided there is adequate evidence for the effectiveness and safety of the treatment. Third, holistic medicine recognizes illness as an imbalance of body systems, similar to the balance of yin/yang principles in Eastern medicine.

Personalized

Any treatment plan needs to be centered on helping to rebuild your health, no matter what tool kit of medicines you draw from. The most successful programs involve a slow-and-steady-wins-the-race approach, like the fable of the tortoise and the hare. Being slow and steady helps you to improve without crashing. We don't want you to yo-yo, like many do with weight-loss plans. We want to see a slow and steady improvement in your ability to function at a high level, one that is sustainable and sets the stage for lifelong balance and health.

Determinants of Good Health

Achieving and maintaining good health is not easy at the best of times, but when you have fibromyalgia, the challenge is even greater. In approaching fibromyalgia, we need to address the various determinants of good health, as defined by the World Health Organization (WHO). These elements determine a person's health, and supporting these elements will help you improve your health.

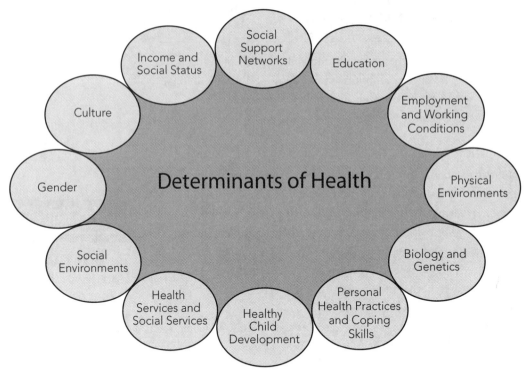

Determinants of Health

Social Support Networks

Income and Social Status

Education

Culture

Employment and Working Conditions

Gender

Physical Environments

Social Environments

Biology and Genetics

Health Services and Social Services

Healthy Child Development

Personal Health Practices and Coping Skills

Courtesy of the World Health Organization.

Patient-Centered

There is a wide variety of strategies that can be used to manage fibromyalgia symptoms. For many of these treatments, you must actively participate in order to receive the maximum benefit. Given the nature of fibromyalgia symptoms — pain, fatigue, brain fog — participation can be a challenge. You will need support from your team of health-care professionals, family, and friends.

Team-Oriented

When we initially see patients at the office, we explain to them that we can often help them improve their symptoms, provided they are willing to play on our team. Managing fibromyalgia is teamwork. We are the team coaches and you are team players. Like any good coach, we are going to ask you to try treatments that will improve your playing ability and your quality of life. If patients want to stay on the team, they will need to try recommended treatments. We do not expect perfection at any visit — only a willingness to try new things as they are suggested. We don't expect patients to master these new skills immediately. Many take time. We do expect you to keep following these therapies. Soon you will notice subtle improvements.

Treatment Goals Worksheet

Start the healing process by setting step-by-step goals, which will keep everything manageable. Don't let the number of the available treatments overwhelm you. Work with your physician or dietitian to set these goals.

Part A: My goals in seeking treatment for my fibromyalgia symptoms are to:

- Improve my current symptoms, functioning, and quality of life
- Feel empowered to trust my own experiences
- Establish supportive therapeutic relationships with my health-care team
- Devise an individualized treatment program
- Learn more about the management of fibromyalgia
- Prevent aggravation of my condition
- Avoid new environment-associated illnesses
- Provide support for my family as everyone adjusts

Part B: Treatments that work to manage fibromyalgia and improve quality of life are not convoluted. They are within your grasp. Check off each treatment systematically as you master these fibromyalgia management strategies:

- Getting a better night's sleep
- Using food as medicine to improve my healing and trying the diet plan in this book
- Empowering myself by learning how to pace activities and rest in between the activities
- Managing pain and other symptoms better
- Learning how to cope with having a chronic illness and the pain of losing your health, your job, and often your friends
- Learning how to clean up your body internally and reduce environmental exposures externally
- Trying new herbs or medications to help improve sleep and reduce pain
- Learning how to grieve the past and find joy in the moment of today
- Taking nutritional supplements if needed
- Learning to balance my yin and yang energy
- Developing an attitude of gratitude to help me find joy in the moment

SEEDS

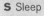

S Sleep

E Energy and Exercise

E Environment

D Diet

S Support

At the Environmental Health Clinic at Women's College Hospital in Toronto, Ontario, Dr. Lynn Marshall and her colleagues have developed a program for improving the quality of life of fibromyalgia patients using a wide variety of strategies that they have grouped under the acronym SEEDS. The aim of this program is to restore homeostasis, or a state of good health. Poor health is the result of the loss of homeostasis, or an imbalance in body systems.

The illustration below shows what happens when a person's life is out of balance. They are overloaded by multiple problems designated as the stressors of health. They suffer from sleep problems, physical weakness from weak muscles, toxicities from environmental exposures, fatigue from a poor diet, and a lack of support to help them with life's daily problems.

Taken together, multiple factors called stressors in this cartoon impact the body systems, leading to an imbalance and eventually resulting in exhaustion.

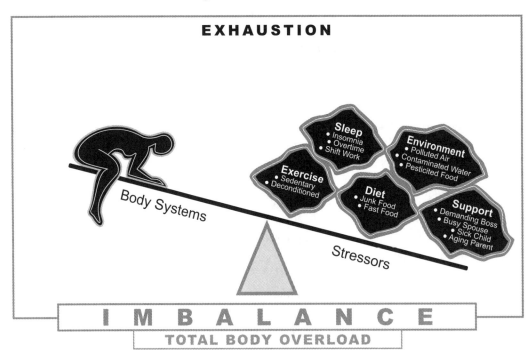

Adapted by permission of Dr. Lynn Marshall, Environmental Health Clinic at Women's College Hospital, Toronto, Ontario.

Sleep

Restorative Sleep

Deep restorative sleep is healing sleep. Sleep is important for normal cognitive (thinking processes) and motor function. Sleep impacts the proper functioning of your organs. Your sleep cycle influences your hormones, your memory, your ability to learn, your digestive function, your metabolism, and even the proper functioning of vital organs, such as your kidneys. Sleep is also important in achieving and maintaining a healthy weight. During sleep, your body secretes hormones that regulate appetite and satiety.

Without deep restorative sleep, your body has difficulty healing. Unfortunately, if you have fibromyalgia, you often do not get enough deep sleep — stage 3 and 4 sleep — as documented in overnight sleep studies. In addition, if your fatigue is compounded by lack of quality sleep, you will be more likely to gravitate toward sugars (simple carbohydrates), which raise blood sugars quickly to provide a quick (but short-lasting) source of energy. Improving the quality of your sleep is essential for healing. Sleep is by its very nature the yin energy that you need to rebuild in order to heal.

| **S Sleep** |
| E Energy and Exercise |
| E Environment |
| D Diet |
| S Support |

Q *What is sleep hygiene?*

A Sleep hygiene is the variety of different practices or routines that are necessary to have the best night sleep you can have. People with fibromyalgia have disrupted sleep. Disrupted deep sleep is a common symptom of fibromyalgia, resulting from body discomfort. If you have fibromyalgia, you likely have trouble finding a comfortable position at night, experience persistent pain, and feel off balance. If you do not wake well rested, you will likely spend the day in a fog, feeling exhausted with continuing body pain. Don't despair … you can improve the quality of your sleep in order to improve your fibromyalgia symptoms. Make sleep hygiene your first step toward recovery.

Tired But Wired

To establish good sleep habits by following natural sleep cycles, you ideally should be in bed by 10:00 p.m. This bedtime is optimal for achieving restorative sleep. If you stay awake beyond this time, you will get your "second wind," which is similar to a runner's high. You end up in a "tired but wired state" because when you get a second wind you get a squirt of endorphins (mood-enhancing chemicals from the brain) that will make you feel good and allow you to stay up for the next couple of hours. When you stay up, you push your body through its fatigued state and end up becoming more fatigued. You are tired physically but wired mentally and cannot sleep afterwards. You are not following your body's natural sleeping rhythm when you do this. You are pushing yourself with false energy and the next morning you will have crashed.

Circadian Rhythms

You sleep in cycles following circadian rhythms, which are the natural 24-hour biological cycles your body follows. Often referred to as the body clock, circadian rhythms are regulated by melatonin and cortisol. These two hormones are involved in regulating your sleep. Melatonin secretion helps you to go to sleep. Secretion starts at 10:00 p.m. as you go to bed and stops at 7:30 a.m. as you wake up. Normally, cortisol levels are highest in the morning to help you handle the day and lowest in the evening after dinner as you start to get ready for bed.

If you fail to follow these natural sleeping and waking cycles, various physical and mental functions are disrupted, including your memory, your ability to learn, your digestive function, your metabolism, and even the proper functioning of your vital organs. Cortisol or melatonin imbalance can aggravate fibromyalgia.

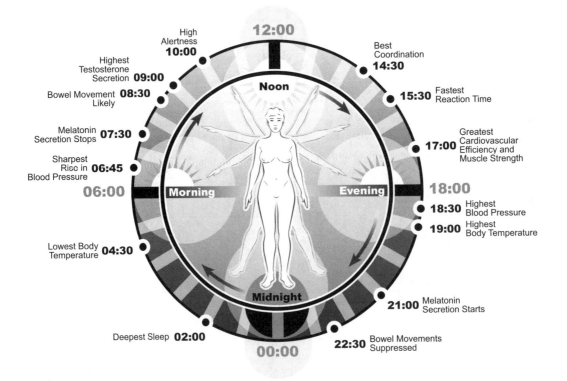

Yoga and Cortisol

In one study of cortisol release in women with fibromyalgia, yoga was shown to raise the levels of cortisol, which in turn reduced pain and improved mindfulness. Mindfulness, which refers to a state of total awareness in the present, is based in Hindu and Buddhist principles. The practice of yoga combines this type of mental meditation with physical movements, stretches, and diaphragmatic breathing techniques to still the body and mind. It also promotes an emotional detachment from external experiences, such as pain, possibly explaining how it works to alleviate psychological symptoms.

Factors Disrupting Cortisol Secretion

- Severe trauma or stressful events elevate cortisol levels.
- Caffeine depresses cortisol secretion.
- Prolonged excessive physical exercise exhausts cortisol.
- Severe calorie restriction elevates cortisol levels.
- Chronic infections or illness lower cortisol levels.
- Depression raises cortisol levels.
- Sleep deprivation disrupts cortisol secretion.

How To Establish a Healthy Sleep Cycle

How you manage your day will directly affect your ability to sleep at night.

- Establish a nighttime routine so you are going to sleep when your body is winding down. Going to bed at 10:00 p.m. and waking 7 to 10 hours later (depending on your body's needs) helps maintain healthy circadian rhythms. If you don't regulate or pace your sleeping hours, you will get a second wind, or an adrenaline rush, and not be able to sleep. The next day, you will have a terrible day and fall into a crashing pattern.
- Do not watch television or use a computer in bed. Watching TV or playing computer games before bedtime is stimulating to your brain and makes it harder to sleep afterward.
- Darken your bedroom with blackout curtains or use a sleep mask at night. This helps the brain to produce the melatonin needed for sleep. In the daytime, surround yourself with bright light so that your brain suppresses melatonin.
- Meditate and relax before bedtime. This helps to increase your parasympathetic state, or the relaxation state of your body, and helps to turn your brain off, allowing you to fall asleep more easily. Meditation also helps you to decrease your

<aside>
Did You Know?

Mindfulness
Scientists believe that yoga promotes a form of mindfulness that is highly effective in the management of pain.
</aside>

pain levels by increasing your body's own pain molecules, called endorphins.

- Take calcium, magnesium, homeopathic remedies, and medications if needed. Drink non-caffeinated herbal teas. These all help the body to relax.
- Make sure your bed is comfortable so that it cushions your body and prevents the worsening of your fibromyalgia pain. Most people like moderate to firm support with a pillow top or eggshell foam on top.

Resetting Your Sleep Clock

If you have become accustomed to going to sleep after 10:00 p.m., you can reverse this trend.

❶ Start by determining what time you are actually falling asleep.
❷ Move bedtime closer to 10:00 p.m. in small, 15-minute increments.
❸ Remember, slow and easy.

For example, if you are getting to bed at midnight but tossing and turning until 2:00 a.m., then 2:00 a.m. is your starting point. In this example, you would then move your bedtime to 1:45 a.m. until you are consistently falling asleep at 1:45 a.m. Once it is consistent, you would move bedtime to 1:30 a.m. and so on, until you are in bed at 10:00 p.m.

Pacing Yourself

Pacing yourself during the day determines if you will be able to fall asleep at night. If you do not pace yourself during the day, by spacing rest periods between your activities, you end up "crashing" by the time you try to go to bed. When you are crashing, you are "tired and wired" — you are physically exhausted but mentally awake. Your overtired brain will likely have a difficult time turning itself off. It is paradoxical, but waiting until you are exhausted before going to bed is not conducive to good-quality sleep. In fact, it almost guarantees that you will toss and turn for hours because your brain cannot turn itself off.

Energy

Energy Conservation

You have a limited amount of energy when you have fibromyalgia. The ability to pace yourself is essential for managing the condition, especially for preventing a flare-up of your symptoms and crashes where you end up exhausted and recovering in bed for hours or days. The goal of pacing is to conserve physical, mental, and emotional energy throughout the day, with the aim of striking a balance between the activities of daily living and resting.

S	Sleep
E	**Energy** and Exercise
E	Environment
D	Diet
S	Support

Look at resting as a healing period that allows your body to recover and to find the energy to begin again once the rest period is finished. Rest means in this case lying down flat on your bed or a supportive couch, with your feet up and your eyes closed. Watching television or reading a book is not resting. Those activities are low-energy activities. If you are not resting, you are not allowing yin (your restorative energy) to rebuild.

Expending Energy

You can "use up" your energy reserves in three ways, but you can use your energy only once:

- **Physically.** For example, you can expend physical energy completing daily activities, such as grocery shopping, house cleaning, and gardening, or working on the job. Despite how simple these physical activities seem, they can exhaust you if you have fibromyalgia and if you don't pace yourself.
- **Mentally.** For example, you can expend mental energy while completing your tax return, budgeting, or solving day-to-day logistics problems created by your fibromyalgia. Brain fog can set in at any time, robbing you of physical energy.
- **Emotionally.** For example, you can expend emotional energy while you feel angry with someone or while you hold a grudge against a friend or family member. However, you can learn to listen to your thoughts and keep them more realistic — instead of exploding in anger or frustration. By keeping your thoughts realistic, you will waste less emotional energy and have more energy available for physical healing.

Physical, Mental, and Emotional Pacing

You can only use your energy once: physically, mentally, or emotionally. Once it is used, it is gone. In this section of the book, the focus is on physical pacing of your body, but pacing also involves mental and emotional energy conservation as you listen to your thoughts and keep your expectations more realistic instead of exploding in anger or frustration. By keeping your thoughts realistic, you will waste less mental and emotional energy and have more energy available for physical healing.

Tools for Learning to Pace Yourself

An activity log is like a daily diary where you keep track of your sleep, activities, rest periods, energy levels, and pain scores. The aim of keeping the activity logs is to learn how to balance your activities and rest periods, and to learn how to pace yourself.

Activity Logs

Activity logs have three functions in the management of fibromyalgia:

❶ First, activity logs can help you see what happens when you pace yourself and when you do not. You can see when you have crashed after an event or activity as a result of trying to do too much or pushing yourself too hard.

❷ Second, activity logs help you plan rest periods in between your activities as a preventive measure so that you do not crash.

❸ Third, activity logs help you respect your body's wisdom. You have learned from experience that it is better to stop than to crash the next day. At this point, you realize that your health is more important than getting more "stuff" done. This is a huge shift in thinking for many patients with fibromyalgia, who in the past have tended to put themselves and their health last.

Components of an Activity Log

An activity log records your sleep duration and quality, your daily activities and rest periods, your energy level (from the functional capacity scale), the number of minutes that you spent walking, and your fibromyalgia symptoms, including your pain level.

Sleep Record

Write down the number of hours you sleep (duration) nightly and quality of your sleep:

1 = very poor • 2 = poor • 3 = fair • 4 = good • 5 = very good

Did You Know?

Activity Log

One way to learn how to pace yourself and practice energy conservation is to complete an activity log on an ongoing basis.

Activity Log

(Feel free to copy this log for your own use. Health-care professionals are welcome to use the log when working with fibromyalgia patients.)

Name: _____ Date Commencing: _____

DAY	Monday	Tuesday	Wednesday	Thursday	Friday	Saturday	Sunday
	6 hrs/3						

Sleep: Record above the number of hours slept and quality
1 = very poor • 2 = poor • 3 = fair • 4 = good • 5 = very good

Activities: Record your daily activities and scheduled exercises below.

Functional Capacity Scale (FCS):
Record your activity and energy rating every hour using the scale 1 to 10

	Monday	Tuesday	Wednesday	Thursday	Friday	Saturday	Sunday
6 a.m.	Meal prep/ FCS 5						
7 a.m.							
8 a.m.							
9 a.m.							
10 a.m.							
11 a.m.							
12 p.m.							
1 p.m.							
2 p.m.							
3 p.m.							
4 p.m.							
5 p.m.							
6 p.m.							
7 p.m.							
8 p.m.							
9 p.m.							
10 p.m.							
11 p.m.							
Exercise: # of minutes walked/day							
# of usable hours/day							

Courtesy of Dr. Alison Bested & Dr. Rosemary Underhill.

If your sleep quality is poor, are you crashing at the end of the day?

Daily Activities Record

In each empty box record your activity; for example, meal preparation, laundry, making a meal. Most patients fill in the boxes with their own shorthand after they have completed a few weeks of activity logs. For example, you would record your rest period as R-20, which means that you rested for 20 minutes. Housework could be HWork, walking could be W-10, which means you walked for 10 minutes. You can write your short forms on the back side of the activity log.

Rest Periods

Write down in the box how many minutes you rested or meditated.

Energy Rating

In each box write down what energy level you were at during that time based on the functional capacity scale. It is most effective if patients record their level of energy hourly so they can see what activities affect their energy.

Time	Monday	Energy Level
8 a.m.	Breakfast, shower	6
9 a.m.	Rest — 20/made beds	5
10 a.m.	Rest — 20/grocery shop 15 minutes	3
11 a.m.	Rest — 60	4
12 a.m.	Lunch	4

Functional Capacity Scale

The functional capacity scale (FCS) incorporates activity level, energy rating, symptom severity, and pain level. The functional capacity scale looks at what you can actually do in terms of functionality both physically and mentally. The description after each scale number should help you to rate your functional capacity hourly throughout the day.

0 = No energy, severe symptoms including very poor concentration; bedridden all day; cannot do self-care (e.g., need bed bath to be given).

1 = Severe symptoms at rest, including very poor concentration; in bed most of the day; need assistance with self-care activities (bathing).

2 = Severe symptoms at rest, including poor concentration; frequent rests or naps; need some assistance with limited self-care activities (can wash face at the sink) and need rest afterward for severe post-exertion fatigue.

3 = Moderate symptoms at rest, including poor concentration; need frequent rests or naps; can do independent self-care (can wash standing at the sink for a few minutes) but have severe post-exertion fatigue and need rest.

4 = Moderate symptoms at rest, including some difficulty concentrating; need frequent rests throughout the day; can do independent self-care (can take a shower) and limited activities of daily living (e.g., light housework, laundry); can walk for a few minutes per day.

5 = Mild symptoms at rest with fairly good concentration for short periods (15 minutes); need a.m. and p.m. rest; can do independent self-care and moderate activities of daily living, but have slight post-exertion fatigue; can walk 10–20 minutes per day.

6 = Mild or no symptoms at rest with fairly good concentration for up to 45 minutes, cannot multitask; need afternoon rest; can do most activities of daily living except vacuuming; can walk 20–30 minutes per day; can do volunteer work — maximum total time 4 hours per week, with flexible hours.

7 = Mild or no symptoms at rest with good concentration for up to ½ day; can do more intense activities of daily living (e.g., grocery shopping, vacuuming) but may get post-exertion fatigue if "overdo": can walk 30 minutes per day; can work limited hours, less than 25 hours per week; no or minimal social life.

8 = Mild intermittent symptoms with good concentration; can do full self-care, work 40 hours per week, enjoy a social life, do moderate vigorous exercise three times per week.

9 = No symptoms with very good concentration, full work and social life; can do vigorous exercise three to five times a week.

10 = No symptoms, excellent concentration, overachiever (sometimes may require less sleep than average person).

NUMBER OF USABLE HOURS/DAY = Number of hours NOT asleep or resting/meditating with eyes closed.

Pain Level

Using the Wong-Baker FACES Pain Rating Scale (page 27), record your level of pain in every box throughout the day so that you can better understand what helps your pain and what activities trigger your pain. This is especially helpful when you are trying a new medication or therapy to see if it is helping reduce your pain levels. Record your pain level, 0 to 10, in a different color ink, such as red so you know that red is your pain level and blue ink is your energy level.

Try using the 0 to 10 visual analog pain scale, with 0 being no pain and 10 being your worst pain.

Other Symptoms

Some patients find it helpful if they record their symptoms and their severities on the back of the activity log to help them determine what activities help or trigger their symptoms.

Fear of Results

Some patients find it difficult to write out and observe how little they can do and are sad to discover how little they actually accomplish in a day. At this point, you may need help, either individually or in a group setting, to deal with the pain and grief of having a chronic illness.

It is most helpful if as you are filling out your logs that you compare yourself to how you were at the worst point in your illness so that you can see how much progress you have made.

It takes practice to accomplish the skill of pacing, so be patient. Your energy levels will begin to even out as you stop crashing. Once you have learned how to pace and avoid crashing, you will see the improvements of your energy over time. Often, months are needed to see improvements.

Guidelines for Keeping an Activity Log

- Change the times on the left-hand side of the log to suit your usual schedule (for example, if you usually get up at 10:00 a.m. and go to bed at 2:00 a.m., write 10:00 a.m. in as the first time cell, and adjust the other times accordingly).
- Note your activities using one or two words or abbreviations in the appropriate time slots (for example, "dressed," "made bed," or "nap").

- Remember that rest is defined as lying down, with your eyes shut, meditating or sleeping.
- Keep your log in a handy place so you can fill it out at any time and complete it every day. Don't try to complete the log at the end of the day. You will not remember what you have done because you have difficulties with your memory.
- Take your completed logs to your doctor or other health-care provider at follow-up visits. Your logs will assist your doctor or other health-care provider determine if your treatment plan needs to be adjusted.
- Hold on to your logs. Completed logs may reassure your insurance company of your active, ongoing participation in your treatment.
- Compare your logs from day to day to learn why you are crashing and how to avoid crashing.
- Compare yourself to how you were at the worst point in your illness so that you can see how much progress you have made.
- Be kind to yourself and patient with your progress. Rome was not built in a day. You will improve gradually, in small increments — baby steps, not giant-size leaps and bounds. Once you have learned how to pace yourself and avoid crashing, you will begin to feel improvements in your energy level.
- Some patients find it helpful to record their symptoms and their severities on a separate page.

Normal Activity Log

This log (see page 51) shows what a normal person's energy levels look like on the activity log. The dark gray means sleep or rest. This person goes to bed at 10:00 p.m. and wakes up at 6:30 a.m. for a total of 8.5 hours sleep. She records that she had great sleep quality — 5 out of 5 — which means she had a good restorative sleep and felt refreshed in the morning when she got up. The white represents normal energy, recorded as 9 to 10 out of 10 on the functional capacity scale. This woman was involved in activities throughout the day, and she did not need any rest periods, as seen by the solid white color throughout the day. Because she had normal energy, she could exercise or walk for 60 minutes four times that week.

Crashing Activity Log

This crashing pattern (see log, page 52) is typical of a patient with fibromyalgia who has not yet learned the way to pace activities and rest. The dark gray means sleep or rest. In this example, she goes to bed at midnight and wakes up at 10:00 a.m. for a total of 10 hours of sleep. She records that she had a sleep quality between 2 and 4 out of 5, which means she had very little restorative sleep on the nights rated at 2, and did not feel refreshed on those mornings. The white represents her normal energy, recorded at 4 to 5 out of 10 on the functional capacity scale at the beginning of the day, and a light gray at the end of the day, where her energy level was 2 to 3 out of 10 on the functional capacity scale. She was able to perform very limited activities throughout the day. However, she did need rest periods, as shown by the dark gray. Because she had very limited energy, she could only exercise or walk for 10 to 20 minutes a few times that week.

Recovery Activity Log

This recovery pattern (see log, page 53) is typical of a patient with fibromyalgia who has learned the way to pace activities and rest. The dark gray means sleep or rest. In this example, she goes to bed at 11:00 p.m. and wakes up at 8:00 a.m. for a total of 9 hours of sleep. She records that she had a sleep quality of 4 out of 5, which means she had some restorative sleep and felt somewhat refreshed in the morning. The white represents her normal energy, which she recorded at 6 out of 10 on the functional capacity scale at the beginning of the day, and a light gray at the end of the day, when her energy level was 5 out of 10 on the functional capacity scale. She was able to perform very limited activities throughout the day — at a higher energy level in the morning and a slightly lower energy level in the afternoon and evening. She regularly scheduled rest periods throughout the day, as shown by the dark gray. As a result of pacing her activities, she could walk for 20 minutes daily.

Normal Activity Log

DAY	Monday	Tuesday	Wednesday	Thursday	Friday	Saturday	Sunday
# of hours slept between 10 p.m. and 6:30 a.m.	8.5/5	8.5/5	8.5/5	8.5/5	8.5/5	8.5/5	8.5/5

Sleep Quality: 1 = very poor • 2 = poor • 3 = fair • 4 = good • 5 = very good

Functional Capacity Scale (FCS): 1 to 10

Activities: Record your daily activities and scheduled exercises below.

	Monday	Tuesday	Wednesday	Thursday	Friday	Saturday	Sunday
6 a.m.							
7 a.m.	9	9	9	9	9	9	9
8 a.m.							
9 a.m.							
10 a.m.							
11 a.m.							
12 p.m.							
1 p.m.							
2 p.m.							
3 p.m.							
4 p.m.							
5 p.m.							
6 p.m.							
7 p.m.							
8 p.m.							
9 p.m.							
10 p.m.							
11 p.m.							
Energy	9	9	9	9	9	9	9
Walked		60		60		60	60

Crashing Activity Log

DAY	Monday	Tuesday	Wednesday	Thursday	Friday	Saturday	Sunday
# of hours slept between 12 p.m. and 10 a.m.	10/4	10/4	10/4	10/2	10/2	10/2	10/3

Sleep Quality: 1 = very poor • 2 = poor • 3 = fair • 4 = good • 5 = very good

Functional Capacity Scale (FCS): 1 to 10

Activities: Record your daily activities and scheduled exercises below.

	Monday	Tuesday	Wednesday	Thursday	Friday	Saturday	Sunday
6 a.m.							
7 a.m.							
8 a.m.							
9 a.m.							
10 a.m.	4	4	5	3	3	3	4
11 a.m.							
12 p.m.							
1 p.m.							
2 p.m.							
3 p.m.							
4 p.m.							
5 p.m.							
6 p.m.							
7 p.m.							
8 p.m.							
9 p.m.							
10 p.m.							
11 p.m.							
Energy	3	3	2	2	2	2	3
Walked	10	10	20	0	0	0	0

Recovery Activity Log

DAY	Monday	Tuesday	Wednesday	Thursday	Friday	Saturday	Sunday
# of hours slept between 11 p.m. and 8 a.m.	9/4	9/4	9/4	9/4	9/4	9/4	9/4

Sleep Quality: 1 = very poor • 2 = poor • 3 = fair • 4 = good • 5 = very good

Functional Capacity Scale (FCS): 1 to 10

Activities: Record your daily activities and scheduled exercises below.

	Monday	Tuesday	Wednesday	Thursday	Friday	Saturday	Sunday
6 a.m.							
7 a.m.							
8 a.m.	6	6	6	6	6	6	6
9 a.m.							
10 a.m.							
11 a.m.							
12 p.m.							
1 p.m.							
2 p.m.							
3 p.m.							
4 p.m.							
5 p.m.							
6 p.m.							
7 p.m.							
8 p.m.							
9 p.m.							
10 p.m.							
11 p.m.							
Energy	5	5	5	5	5	5	5
Walked	20	20	20	20	20	20	20

Crashing vs. Recovering Activity Patterns

Crashing Characteristics	Recovering Characteristics
Ignores the body's signals	Listens to the body's signals
Puts health last	Puts health first
Does not know their limits	Knows their limits
Wants to please others (people pleaser)	Feels comfortable saying no to others (sets boundaries)
Pushes themselves to get things done	Paces themselves to get things done
Has many demanding/toxic people in their life	Has chosen supportive people and eliminated toxic people from their life
Denies they have a chronic illness	Understands their illness and is actively managing it
Has rock-and-roll energy with no ability to plan ahead	Has learned to manage their energy and now can plan ahead and manage activities

Regimens

Patients who fare the best tend to be regimented about completing their activity logs and functional capacity reports. This regimen is especially important during times when you are improving and may think you do not need to complete your logs and scales. But these logs can prevent you from falling back into old patterns of pushing too hard — only to later suffer the devastating effects of a crash.

Exercise

Exercise Programs

S Sleep

E Energy and **Exercise**

E Environment

D Diet

S Support

The aim of keeping the activity logs is to allow you to stay as active as possible without crashing and suffering from a major flare-up and to gradually build muscle and bone to prevent osteoporosis. This principle of doing things gradually applies to any exercise programs you may adopt. Introduce formal exercise programs into your life very slowly, and consider the kind of exercise that is best for your symptoms. It is recommended that you be assessed by a professional, such as a physiotherapist or someone who understands muscle function, before you begin any exercise program.

Kinds of Exercise

There are several kinds of exercise that can be employed in managing fibromyalgia, but all exercise regimens need to be "backed off" in intensity for the fibromyalgia patient to handle according to her individual needs.

Range-of-Motion and Stretching Exercises

Range-of-motion exercises (also called stretching or flexibility exercises) keep the muscles and joints flexible and as strong as possible even if a patient is bedbound. In this group of exercises, gently straightening and bending the joints in a controlled manner as far as they comfortably will go can help condition the affected joints. During the course of a range-of-motion exercise program, the joints are stretched progressively farther until a normal or near-normal range is achieved and maintained. This helps to maintain comfort while function is preserved.

Passive range-of-motion exercises can be done for the patient by a caregiver. Active range-of-motion exercises are done by the patient and can be done even while in bed. If you are in bed, ask if a physiotherapist can come to your home to get you started. Use a soothing massage to begin warming the joints and increasing the muscle circulation, or apply mild heat to the muscles and joints, before beginning the exercises.

Resistance and Strengthening Exercises

Strong muscles help keep weak joints stable and protect them against further damage. A program of strengthening exercises that targets specific muscle groups can be helpful as part of your fibromyalgia treatment. Strengthening exercises, when performed properly, can maintain or increase muscle tissue to support your muscles without aggravating your joints. These exercises use your own body weight or external weights to increase muscle strength. They include aqua therapy, resistance bands, free weights, and weight machines.

You need professional guidance to begin these exercises. Most patients with fibromyalgia enjoy going to aqua therapy classes more than other exercise programs because the classes are held in warm water-pools with other people who have fibromyalgia or arthritis. Being in the water means adding resistance training (from moving against the water), but spares pressure on the joints because the water supports your body. People often exercise in comfort and they form support networks with the people they exercise with.

Fatigue

Most patients with fibromyalgia have difficulty with fatigue after exercise, so again you need the help of a professional to guide you so that you do not overdo your capacity and crash after you exercise.

Arm and Leg Raises

Arm and leg raises combine the qualities of range-of-motion exercises and resistance exercises. They are low impact and can be practiced every day. These should be done with the guidance of a physiotherapist. Only do what you can manage without crashing.

❶ Slowly raise an arm or leg up and lower it slowly back to the bed. Do this for a total of 90 seconds maximum when you begin exercising if you are bedridden. Start slowly with any new exercise activity so you can keep on doing it in the long run. Begin by doing these exercises two times a week to give your body time to recover in between.

❷ Work up to 2 sets of 8 raises as you are able without pushing yourself and with no crashing afterward.

❸ Slowly mobilize out of bed to regain your abdominal strength. Use a walker or canes if your balance is unsteady. If you are in a wheelchair you can begin to do some modified arm and leg exercises while you are sitting in your wheelchair.

Aerobic Exercise

Aerobic exercise is sustained exercise that increases blood flow to the muscles, strengthening the cardiovascular system and lungs in the presence of oxygen. Maximum benefits are achieved when an aerobic activity is performed for at least 30 minutes per day in total. It can be spread out in small segments of time throughout the day to suit your energy level, without overexerting yourself.

Aerobic exercise should be performed at a comfortable, steady pace that allows you to talk normally and easily during the activity. Ask your therapist which intensity of exercise is appropriate for your fitness level.

Aerobic Choices

Examples of aerobic activities include walking, swimming, low-impact aerobic dance, skiing, and biking, as well as such daily activities as mowing the lawn, raking leaves, and playing golf. Walking is one of the easiest aerobic exercises; it requires no special skills or equipment other than a good pair of supportive walking shoes, and it is less stressful on joints than running or jogging.

Biking is another good choice for people with fibromyalgia because it places less stress on knee, foot, and ankle joints. Biking on a stationary bike or adult tricycle works well for people with FM because they have difficulties with balance. Biking on a regular bicycle for most fibromyalgia patients is not recommended because of their poor balance and slower speed of processing information mentally, which makes it more likely they will have a bike accident. Swimming is also often recommended because there is minimal pressure on joints while in water.

Exercise Rules
- Make sure to increase your level of exercise slowly; use the 10% rule. If you can walk 10 minutes daily, and on a good day you want to walk more, you can increase your walking by 10%, which is an increase of 1 minute more for a total of 11 minutes of walking.
- Always warm up before exercise and stretch afterward.
- Try strength training with slow movements to prevent osteoporosis.
- Choose low-impact exercises, such as water exercise.

---

10 Tips for Beginning Any Exercise Program

Before starting any exercise program, be sure to meet with an exercise and activity professional, such as a physiotherapist or osteopath, who understands muscle function.

1. Start where you are right now with your illness. If you are in bed, ask if a physiotherapist can come to your home to get you started.
2. If you are confined to a bed, start with range-of-motion exercises. This means moving your arms, legs, and body in the directions it can normally move. For example, the arm can move in a circle — side to side and front to back. The legs can be raised and lowered.
3. Exercise initially for 90 seconds maximum.
4. Chart your progress on your activity log.
5. Monitor your heart rate while doing your exercises. If your heart rate rises above the aerobic threshold or if you feel like you are overexerting yourself, back off and rest or meditate (feet up and eyes closed).
6. Walk between the benches. If you can walk on a good day but crash afterward, you are likely walking more than your body can manage at one time. Try walking the same distance but breaking it up into smaller bits with rests in between. Some patients call this "walking between the benches." Walking at an inside mall is great for this concept.

7 Increase your exercise activity slowly. If you think you can do more on a good day, increase by only 10% so you don't crash later. Slow and steady wins this race.

8 If you have been inactive, you run the risk of developing osteoporosis (melting bones). To avoid this, exercise with resistance bands or weights. Community centers often offer osteoporosis exercise programs on land or in pools.

9 Start initially with no weights to condition your muscles in this new exercise. When you do add resistance use a flex band or try only one exercise using a half-pound (250 g) weight and do only 3 repetitions. If you do too much too fast, you run the risk of injury to your tendons and ligaments.

10 Do your exercises under the supervision of a professional if possible.

Environment

Environmental Exposures

S Sleep

E Energy and Exercise

E **Environment**

D Diet

S Support

The seeds of good health will not grow if the soil is contaminated. To manage fibromyalgia, you will need to reduce, if not eliminate, the various toxins in your internal and external environments that can trigger your illness. This process of detoxification means looking at a variety of exposures, including exposure to heavy metals, that may have accumulated in your body. Other exposures include pesticides, food additives, and polluted air, soil, and water.

Chemical Exposure Questionnaire

At the Environmental Health Clinic at Women's College Hospital in Toronto, Dr. Lynn Marshall and her colleagues have developed a questionnaire to help determine your possible exposure to toxins and your possible level of contamination. This environmental history helps your doctor ascertain all the potential sources of toxins. Complete the Community, Home, Hobbies, Occupation, Personal Habits, Diet, and Drugs (CH^2OPD^2) Assessment.

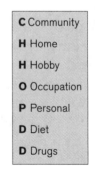

C Community

H Home

H Hobby

O Occupation

P Personal

D Diet

D Drugs

Taking an Exposure History

The mnemonic CH^2OPD^2 helps to organize the patient's history, and the questionnaire can be given to patients to be completed at home and reviewed at a subsequent educational counseling visit.

Exposure History

❶ Community

Do you presently live near any of the following?

YEARS

Heavy traffic ☐ No ☐Yes (please specify) ☐ Highway ☐ Busy street   ___

Vehicle idling area ☐ No ☐Yes (please specify) ☐ Auto ☐ Bus/truck   ___

Dump site ☐ No ☐ Yes (please specify type)_____ ___

Farm(s) ☐ No ☐ Yes (please specify type)_____ ___

Industrial plants ☐ No ☐Yes (please specify type)_____ ___

Polluted lake/stream ☐ No ☐ Yes (please specify type) _____ ___

Nuclear power plant ☐ No ☐ Yes _____ ___

Electricity towers ☐ No ☐ Yes _____ ___

Cell phone towers ☐ No ☐ Yes _____ ___

Windmills or turbines ☐ No ☐ Yes _____ ___

Other potential hazards ☐ No ☐ Yes (please specify type) _____ ___

Do you protect yourself from excess sun exposure? How? _____ ___

☐ Rarely ☐ Occasionally ☐ Often ☐ Always

❷ Home and Hobby

How long have you lived in your present residence? _____ How old is it? _____

What type of dwelling is your residence?

☐ Detached house ☐ Semi-detached house ☐ Mobile home ☐ Apartment

☐ Basement ☐ Above a store ☐ High or low rise

☐ Number of floors _____ ☐ Your floor _____

Do you rent or own? ☐ Owner occupied ☐ Rental ☐ Co-op ☐ Public housing

How is your home heated?

☐ Forced air ☐ Hot water radiators ☐ Space heater ☐ Baseboard heaters

What type of fuel is used for heating?

☐ Natural gas ☐ Oil ☐ Wood ☐ Electricity ☐ Propane

What kind of vacuum do you use? ☐ Central vacuum ☐ HEPA filter vacuum

☐ Other vacuum (please specify type) _____

Do you use any of these electronics?

☐ Cell phone ☐ Cordless phone ☐ Laptop computer

Have you done any renovating? ☐ No ☐ Yes ☐ When?_____

What did you renovate? _____

Do you own/lease a car? ☐ No ☐ Yes ☐ Age _____

Is smoking permitted inside? ☐ No ☐ Yes

Adapted by permission of Dr. Lynn Marshall, Environmental Health Clinic at Women's College Hospital, Toronto, Ontario.

Do you use pesticides or herbicides (bug or weed killers, flea/tick sprays, collars, powders, pellets, etc.)?

(1) In the home ☐ No ☐ Yes (please specify type) _____

(2) On pets ☐ No ☐ Yes (please specify type) _____

(3) On the lawn or garden ☐ No ☐ Yes (please specify type)_____

Does anyone in your household use these on the job?

☐ Pesticide ☐ Strong chemicals (please specify type) _____

What is your water source for bathing? ☐ City ☐ Well

☐ Other (please specify) _____

Do you presently have any of the following in your home? If you had one of these things in the past, note the years at right.

Basement cracks or dirt floor ☐ No ☐ Yes (circle one or both)

Crawl space ☐ No ☐ Yes (circle one or both)

Damp, musty basement ☐ No ☐ Yes (circle one or both)

Wet windows or outside closet walls (condensation) ☐ No ☐ Yes ☐ Slight ☐ Severe

Water leaks ☐ No ☐ Yes ☐ Slight ☐ Severe Where? _____

Visible mold ☐ No ☐ Yes ☐ Slight ☐ Severe Where? _____

Crumbling pipe insulation ☐ No ☐ Yes ☐ Slight ☐ Severe

Flaking paint ☐ No ☐ Yes ☐ Slight ☐ Severe

Stagnant, stuffy air ☐ No ☐ Yes ☐ Slight ☐ Severe

Gas or propane stove ☐ No ☐ Yes (circle one or both)

Other gas appliances ☐ No ☐ Yes (please specify) _____

Wood stove or fireplace ☐ No ☐ Yes (circle one or both)

Carbon monoxide detector(s) ☐ No ☐ Yes Where? _____

Air conditioning ☐ No ☐ Yes ☐ Central ☐ Individual rooms

Electrostatic air cleaner ☐ No ☐ Yes

Other air cleaner(s) ☐ No ☐ Yes (please specify) _____

Carpets ☐ No ☐ Yes

Where? (e.g., basement, bedroom) _____

How old? _____

Old vinyl linoleum ☐ No ☐ Yes

Computer(s) ☐ No ☐ Yes Where? _____

Wireless? ☐ No ☐ Yes

Photocopier/fax machine/printer ☐ No ☐ Yes Where? _____

Garage ☐ No ☐ Yes ☐ Attached ☐ Underground

Smoker(s) ☐ No ☐ Yes Who? _____

Pets ☐ No ☐ Yes (please specify kind and number) _____

Pets sleep in your bedroom ☐ No ☐ Yes (please specify) _____

Indoor plants ☐ No ☐ Yes How many?_____

Do you use an electric blanket? ☐ No ☐ Yes

Do you use a bedside electric clock and/or radio? ☐ No ☐ Yes

Do you use dust mite-proof bedding? Pillow cover(s) ☐ No ☐ Yes

Mattress cover(s) ☐ No ☐ Yes

Age of your mattress _____

What hobbies do you have?_____

Have you ever personally done any of the following?

☐ Furniture stripping/refinishing

☐ Home renovating (please specify type) _____

☐ Art work (e.g., painting, ceramics, stained glass, leatherwork)

(please specify type)   _____

☐ Other non-occupational activities with exposure to toxic chemicals

(please specify type)   _____

What product(s) and brand(s) do you usually use?

Bathroom cleanser _____ Floor/wall cleanser _____

Window cleaner _____

Laundry detergent _____ Fabric softener_____ Air freshener _____

❸ Occupation

A. Do you presently do volunteer work and/or work for pay? ☐ No ☐ Yes

If yes,	☐ Volunteer work ☐ Number of hours per week _____ Type _____
	☐ Work for pay ☐ Number of hours per week _____
If no,	☐ Unable to work for pay due to health problems Date stopped work _____ Reason(s) _____ ☐ On disability benefits ☐ Type _____ OR ☐ Disability claim ☐ Unresolved ☐ Permanently denied

B. Starting with your present or most recent job, please list all of the paying jobs you have ever had (including summer jobs). Please use additional paper if necessary.

Company name and work location	From month/year	To month/year	Job title and description	Exposures*	Protective measures/ equipment**
1.	/	/			
2.	/	/			
3.	/	/			
4.	/	/			

Please list the significant chemicals, dusts, fibers, fumes, ionizing radiation, electromagnetic fields, biological agents (e.g., bacteria, molds, viruses), and physical agents (e.g., extreme heat, cold, vibration, noise) that you were exposed to at this job.

** *Please list any protective measures taken (e.g., showering at work, laundering clothes at work) or protective equipment used (e.g., gloves, apron, mask, respirator, hearing protectors, shield) at this job.*

C. The following questions relate to your present or most recent work environment.
Age of building _____ Number of floors _____ Approximate number of occupants _____
Neighborhood: ☐ Rural ☐ Commercial ☐ Industrial
Which of the following are/were on the same floor as your workstation or work environment?
☐ Wi-Fi ☐ Banks of computers
☐ Partitions or room dividers ☐ Unvented copy machines
☐ Unvented smoking areas ☐ Carpets ☐ How old?_____
☐ Co-workers complaining of feeling ill at work
Please specify symptoms _____
☐ Central air conditioning ☐ Windows that open ☐ Number? _____
Can/could you smell any of these odors in your work environment? ☐ Laboratory
☐ Cafeteria ☐ Manufacturing area ☐ Idling vehicles ☐ Parking garage
Have any of the following occurred over the past 12 months or during the last
12 months you worked in your most recent job?
☐ Use of pesticides ☐ Indoors ☐ Outdoors
☐ Fire/smoke ☐ Flood/water leaks ☐ Carpet cleaning
☐ New flooring, furniture, etc. (please specify) _____
☐ Construction ☐ Renovation
☐ Painting ☐ Chemical spill/leaks (please specify) _____
☐ Accidents ☐ Stress
On average, how would you describe your work environment in terms of the following conditions?
Lighting ☐ Too much glare ☐ Satisfactory ☐ Too dim
Temperature ☐ Too hot ☐ Satisfactory ☐ Too cold ☐ Too variable
Air movement ☐ Too stuffy ☐ Satisfactory ☐ Too drafty
Humidity ☐ Too dry ☐ Satisfactory ☐ Too humid
Odor ☐ None ☐ Moderate ☐ Strong (please specify) _____
Noise ☐ Little ☐ Moderate ☐ A lot
Your comfort overall ☐ Unsatisfactory ☐ Somewhat satisfactory ☐ Satisfactory
Co-workers' comfort overall
☐ Unsatisfactory ☐ Somewhat satisfactory ☐ Satisfactory

❹ **School**
☐ Not applicable
How old is your (or your child's) school? _____ Number of floors _____
Approximate number of occupants _____

Have additions been made to the original building? ☐ No ☐ Yes ☐ When? _____

Number of portable classrooms in use _____

Hours daily you or your child spends in a portable classroom _____

School neighborhood: ☐ Rural ☐ Suburban ☐ Urban

Is your (or your child's) school located near any of the following?

Heavy traffic ☐ No ☐ Yes (please specify) ☐ Highway ☐ Busy street

Vehicle idling area ☐ No ☐ Yes (please specify) ☐ Auto ☐ Bus/truck

Dump site ☐ No ☐ Yes (please specify)_____

Farm(s) ☐ No ☐ Yes (please specify) _____

Industrial plant(s) ☐ No ☐ Yes (please specify) _____

Polluted lake/stream ☐ No ☐ Yes (please specify)_____

Nuclear power plant ☐ No ☐ Yes_____

Electricity towers ☐ No ☐ Yes _____

Other potential hazards ☐ No ☐ Yes (please specify type)_____

Which of the following does your (or your child's) school have? Please check all that apply.

☐ Computers ☐ Wi-Fi ☐ Carpeted classrooms ☐ Central air conditioning

☐ Art room — exhaust hood? ☐ No ☐ Yes ☐ Unvented copy machine(s)

☐ Windows that open ☐ Laboratory — exhaust hood? ☐ No ☐ Yes

☐ Flaking paint ☐ Moldy smell ☐ Workshop — exhaust hood? ☐ No ☐ Yes

Have any of the following occurred in your (or your child's) school during the current or last school year?

Please check all that apply.

☐ Carpet cleaning ☐ Construction ☐ Renovations ☐ Painting ☐ Roof tarring

☐ New flooring or furniture (please specify) _____

☐ Flood/water leaks ☐ Use of pesticides/herbicides ☐ Indoors ☐ Outdoors

Are the following products used in your (or your child's) school during the school year?

☐ Deodorizer strips ☐ Furniture wax or polish ☐ Odorous cleaning products

☐ Deodorant sprays ☐ Floor wax ☐ Scented washroom soap

☐ Spray paints ☐ Permanent markers ☐ Strong-smelling art supplies

Does your (or your child's) school have a policy regarding the use of personal scented products by staff and students?

☐ No ☐ Yes (please specify) ☐ Prohibition of scented products

☐ Encouragement of unscented products

❺ Personal

Natural Inhalant Allergies

Do you think you are allergic to any seasonal pollens, animal danders, dustmites, or molds?

☐ No ☐ Yes (please specify) _____

Have you ever had allergy tests? ☐ No ☐ Yes If yes, please specify:

Age	Year	Type of test	Results	Treatments (e.g., avoidance, shots, medications)	Improvement 0 = worse 1 = none 2 = little 3 = some 4 = a lot

Synthetic Chemicals

Have you ever had symptoms that you linked* to the exposure** of any synthetic (man-made) chemical at a level that did not seem to bother most people (e.g., paints, perfumes, cosmetics, diesel exhaust, jet fuel, tar)? ☐ No ☐ Yes

* *"Linked" means that the symptoms started or worsened within 48 hours after you were exposed to something or that the symptom improved or disappeared after you were no longer exposed to it.*

** *"Exposure" means being near, touching, smelling, breathing in, eating, drinking, swallowing, or injecting something.*

If yes, please specify:

Man-made chemical	Symptoms linked with low-level exposure	Presently affected? 1 = a little 2 = somewhat 3 = a lot	In the past? 1 = a little 2 = somewhat 3 = a lot

How often do you use scented personal products? Please check all that apply.

	Never	Occasionally	Daily
Scented products			
Other soap			
Lotion			
Cosmetics			
Hair dye (permanent)			
Hair tint			
Perfume/aftershave (please specify)			

Artificial Materials and Electromagnetic Fields

How many metal dental fillings/crowns/caps do you currently have?

Silver/mercury _____ Gold _____

Have you had silver/mercury fillings removed? ☐ No ☐ Yes

Number removed _____ Year(s) _____

Do you have other artificial materials in your body (e.g., pins, screws, plates, meshes, valves, implants)? ☐ No ☐ Yes (please specify) _____

Have you ever thought you were allergic or very sensitive to electrical appliances, computers, or power lines? ☐ No ☐ Yes (please specify)_____

Smoking History

Do you currently use tobacco (daily or almost every day)?

☐ No ☐ Yes (please specify) ☐ Cigarettes ☐ Cigars ☐ Pipe
☐ Snuff ☐ Chewing tobacco

If yes, average number per day _____ Number of years_____

Interested in a smoking-cessation program? ☐ Yes ☐ No

Date you last used tobacco regularly _____

Have you been exposed to secondhand smoke daily or almost every day?

☐ No ☐ Yes Number of years _____

Have you ever experimented with recreational drugs? ☐ No ☐ Yes

List names of drugs and time used _____

❻ Travel Illnesses

Have you ever experienced significant symptoms when travelling? ☐ No ☐ Yes
If yes, please specify.

Age	Year	Location	Symptoms

Do you recall having tick bite(s)? ☐ No ☐ Yes ☐ If yes, when? _____
Where? _____
Do you recall having a bull's-eye-like rash around an insect bite? ☐ No ☐ Yes
When? _____ Where? _____

❼ Living Situation/Supports

Who lives at home with you? _____

What is your marital status?

☐ Single ☐ Married/cohabitating ☐ Separated ☐ Divorced ☐ Widowed

How do you feel about your living situation? ☐ Happy ☐ Unhappy

Do you have spiritual beliefs/practices that help you cope?

☐ No ☐ Yes (please comment) _____

Are you part of a religious community that helps you cope?

☐ No ☐ Yes (please estimate the number of contacts in the last 12 months) _____

Who best supports you with your present health problems? _____

What other supports do you have? _____

❽ Stresses

Type of stress	Ever experienced it?	When? (Please specify year)	Comments
Loss of someone close	☐ No ☐ Yes		
Illness in someone close	☐ No ☐ Yes		
Loss of job	☐ No ☐ Yes		
Change of job	☐ No ☐ Yes		
Change of workplace	☐ No ☐ Yes		
A move	☐ No ☐ Yes		
Marriage	☐ No ☐ Yes		
Separation	☐ No ☐ Yes		
Divorce	☐ No ☐ Yes		
Pregnancy	☐ No ☐ Yes		
Alcohol/drug addiction	☐ No ☐ Yes		
Alcohol/drug addiction in someone close	☐ No ☐ Yes		
Physical abuse	☐ No ☐ Yes		
Emotional abuse (e.g., being put down, called names)	☐ No ☐ Yes		
Sexual abuse	☐ No ☐ Yes		
Other (please specify)	☐ No ☐ Yes		

❾ Diet and Drugs

A. Who grocery shops for you? _____

Where? ☐ Chain grocery store ☐ Health food store ☐ Market ☐ Online

☐ Other (please specify) _____

B. Who cooks for you? _____

C. Please indicate foods and beverages most typically consumed for each of the following meals and the times at which they are most typically eaten.

Foods/snacks	Please specify	Time	Beverage(s)	Please specify	Time
Breakfast			Breakfast		
Mid-morning			Mid-morning		
Lunch			Lunch		
Mid-afternoon			Mid-afternoon		
Dinner			Dinner		
Evening			Evening		

D. How much of the following beverages do you consume regularly, and have you linked any symptoms with drinking them?

☐ Water ☐ Number of 8-oz (250 mL) glasses per 24 hours _____

☐ City ☐ Charcoal-filtered ☐ Distilled

☐ Reverse-osmosis ☐ Bottled (glass) ☐ Bottled (plastic)

Any symptoms linked? _____

☐ Beer/ale ☐ Number of 12-oz (341 mL) bottles per week _____

Any symptoms linked? _____

☐ Wine ☐ Number of 6-oz (175 mL) glasses per week _____

Any symptoms linked? _____

☐ Spirits (e.g., whisky, rum) ☐ Number of $1\frac{1}{2}$-oz (45 mL) drinks per week _____

Any symptoms linked? _____

☐ Coffee ☐ Number of 8-oz (250 mL) cups per 24 hours_____

Any symptoms linked? _____

☐ Tea ☐ Number of 8-oz cups (250 mL) per 24 hours _____

Any symptoms linked? _____

☐ Cola ☐ Number of 12-oz (375 mL) drinks per 24 hours _____

☐ Regular ☐ Diet Any symptoms linked?_____

Other(s) (please specify) _____

Any symptoms linked? _____

E. Do you eat fish or seafood? ☐ No ☐ Yes

On average, how many days per week? _____

How many times per day? _____

Types of fish or seafood eaten (e.g., tuna, salmon, shrimps, oysters) _____

F. Do you use artificial sweetener? ☐ No ☐ Yes

On average, how many days per week? _____

How many times per day? _____ Type(s) of sweetener _____

G. Please list foods and beverages that do not agree with you (e.g., stuffy/
   runny nose, heartburn, bloating, diarrhea, sleepiness, difficulty thinking/
   concentrating) or cause allergic reactions (e.g., hives, rashes, shortness of breath,
   wheezing, anaphylaxis).

List foods/ beverages that are a problem	What problem(s) do they give you?	Approximately how often do you eat/drink them?			
		Never	Occasionally	Daily	More than once a day

H. Please list any foods and beverages that you crave or that help you to feel better,
   and the time(s) of day the craving usually occurs.

List foods/ beverages that you crave or that help you to feel better	Time(s) of craving	What problem(s) do they give you?	Approximately how often do you eat/drink them?		
			Never	Occasionally	Daily

I. Please list all prescription medications you currently take on a regular basis,
    including birth control pills and allergy injections (use additional paper
    if necessary).

Name of prescription medication	Dose (e.g., mg, mL, IU)	How often do you take it?	How long have you taken it?	If you have side effects, please specify	For office use only

J. Please list all non-prescription medications you currently take on a regular basis, including vitamins, minerals, herbs, remedies, etc. (use additional paper if necessary).

Name and brand of non-prescription medication	Dose (e.g., mg, mL, IU)	How often do you take it?	How long have you taken it?	If you have side effects, please specify	For office use only

K. Have you experienced any drug-adverse reactions? Please list any medication/
anesthetic/immunization you have had to stop taking because of side effects or
allergic reactions.

Name of medication/ anesthetic/ immunization	Type of side effects or allergic reaction that caused you to stop taking it	Age	Year

L. Have you ever had an emergency injection of adrenaline (epinephrine) for a
reaction to any medication, food, insect sting, or other substance?

☐ No ☐ Yes What year(s)? _____

To what? _____

Environmental Inventory

Use this exposure questionnaire to make a list of toxins you remember being exposed to. No one knows for certain the degree to which these exposures affect people. Since World War II, 70,000 new chemicals have been created, and fewer than 10,000 have been assessed for short- or long-term human health problems.

Heavy Metal Poisoning

Exposure to mercury can be caused by the consumption of large cold-water fish (tuna, swordfish, and shark, for example) or from the mercury used in dental amalgams. Exposure to aluminum could be from antiperspirants, food, or water. Routes of exposure to heavy metals include inhaling, injecting, ingesting, and absorbing through your skin. Toxins are naturally removed from the body through the liver system, so supporting liver function is essential. Once environmental triggers are identified, the goal is to avoid, reduce, and remove them.

Detoxification

Several strategies have been developed for detoxifying, cleansing, and ridding the body of this chemical load besides supporting your liver with clean food and water. Chelation and therapeutic saunas have proven to be effective. Some herbs are also used in heavy metal detoxification, such as chlorella and *Coriandrum sativum*.

Chelation Therapy

Chelation is used as a treatment for acute heavy metal poisoning, including mercury, iron, arsenic, and lead. The chelating agent or medication may be administered orally, intramuscularly, or intravenously, depending on the agent and the type of poisoning. Heavy metal detoxification may be helpful if you have a history of exposure to such toxins as mercury and aluminum.

Caution and medically guided supervision need to be in place before doing any sort of chelation to ascertain whether you are carrying a heavy metal burden and before embarking on any sort of heavy metal detoxification program, such as chelation. Heavy metal detoxification should be done under the supervision of a professional with specific training in this kind of detoxification.

Infrared Sauna

Infrared saunas can be used to enhance the detoxification process. The saunas have been shown to decrease oxidative

> **Common Toxins and Examples**
> - Biological agents (mold in our homes)
> - Inorganic chemicals (arsenic in our groundwater)
> - Organic chemicals (household cleaners)
> - Electromagnetic fields (cell phones)
> - Viruses (contagious people)
> - Emotional ("toxic" people)

stress, improve circulation, and increase sweating, which eliminates toxins through the pores. All sauna programs should be medically supervised at first. Limit time in the sauna to a few minutes at a time initially to be sure you can tolerate the process. Saunas are usually well tolerated. A cooler shower is recommended following the sauna. You can work up to do a series of three 15-minute cycles in the sauna followed by a 30-second to 1-minute cooler shower.

Alka Powder Supplement

To enhance the effect of the sauna, use an alkaline powder.

❶ Start by drinking a mixture of $\frac{1}{4}$ teaspoon (1 mL) of alka powder (sodium bicarbonate) or Alka Seltzer Gold tablets in an 8 oz glass of water prior to starting the sauna.

❷ Take into the sauna 1 teaspoon (5 mL) of alka powder mixed into 4 cups (1 L) of water to drink while you are in the sauna. Alka powder is available in power or capsules and contains a balanced combination of citric acid, potassium bicarbonate and sodium bicarbonate to help replace salts when you are sweating and restore your alkaline/acidic pH balance.

Caution: Do not take alka powder it if you are on a potassium- or sodium-restricted diet or have kidney disease. Stop the sauna if you feel dizzy or confused and experience muscle spasms or cramping.

Diet

S Sleep

E Energy and Exercise

E Environment

D Diet

S Support

Poor diet can trigger fibromyalgia and prevent recovery if not corrected. However, changing your eating habits is one of the most difficult changes in behavior you will make while working to manage your fibromyalgia symptoms because food is a source of emotional support as well as a physical need. Many people eat when they are sad, mad, lonely, or just plain bored. Before you eat, ask yourself, "Am I eating because my body needs to eat or am I eating to help with my emotions?" If you are eating for emotional reasons, try to find an alternative way to deal with your upset feelings. Then ask yourself, "Is this food building or depleting me?" If the answer is that it is depleting you, make sure you make a big deposit on the building side to compensate. Once you have planted the seeds that build and nurture you, make sure to continue to feed them. This is a lifelong journey, not a quick fix. You need to ensure your life going forward is one of balance, where the seeds are always fed.

Refreshed Diet

Much of this book is devoted to guiding you in selecting refreshing foods that do not trigger fibromyalgia and in preparing anti-fibromyalgia meals. For now, start by changing your eating habits.

- Don't forget to eat (especially breakfast).
- Eat three meals daily, plus one or two snacks.
- Avoid known food sensitivities and allergies.
- Drink 8 to 10 glasses of water or other fluids daily. That is equivalent to 64 ounces (2 L).
- Eat organic whole foods with no chemical additives or preservatives if you can afford to.
- Consult a health-care professional before taking nutritional supplements.
- View food as medicine, absolutely necessary for good health.

Support

Stress Reduction

As a result of having a chronic illness, you need support. Ideally, this can come from your family and friends. You need support to deal with your physical illness and also to deal with the emotional impact of having a chronic illness that has robbed you of your health, your livelihood, and your self-esteem. At some stage in your healing process, you will need to identify, acknowledge, and begin to remove any obstacles to your healing or stressors that are depleting you of your energy. Stress can worsen fibromyalgia symptoms. Stressors may come from a variety of sources, including work, friends, family, and your environment.

To lower your stress level, you can start by identifying sources of stress. Consider external stressors, such as family or work demands, and internal stressors, such as financial stress from being on a disability pension and learning how to live on 40% less income. Next, seek out effective strategies for coping with stress, including an anti-inflammatory diet, massage therapy, aqua therapy, meditation, counseling, and mind-body strategies.

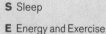

S Sleep

E Energy and Exercise

E Environment

D Diet

S Support

Q *What is stress?*

A Contrary to popular opinion, stress is not "just in your head." In fact, stress is translated by your endocrine system into your body organs by using the body's biochemistry. It is real, with a clear pathology involving the hypothalamus-pituitary-adrenal axis and the adrenal hormone cortisol. Stress is what you experience when you feel under attack, known as the flight or fight response. It is the feeling when you feel unable to cope with specific challenges in your life. Stress can be acute (short term) or chronic (long term). In the short term, acute stress may have beneficial effects in protecting you against physical injury. This is the fight or flight response. If you run into a grizzly bear while hiking in the mountains, this response will help you to flee — or to stand and fight if flight is not possible. In the long term, chronic stress will deplete your energy, leading to fatigue and exhaustion. Over time, even moderate levels of stress can have serious health consequences.

The result of prolonged stress is exhaustion. Fibromyalgia symptoms worsen with exhaustion, which occurs when you crash.

Stress Inventory

Stress can impede your effort to manage the symptoms of fibromyalgia. Taking an inventory of the stressors in your life is one step forward to recovery. Your health-care provider can help you set goals for reducing stress and provide practical therapies.

❶ Make a list of the top 10 stressors in your life.
❷ Rate each stressor from 1 to 5, with 1 being an occasional annoyance and 5 being almost unbearable anxiety.
❸ Explore the source of the stressor and target a possible solution.
❹ Once you complete reading this section of the book on fibromyalgia treatments, come back to this inventory and see if your stressors are less severe. Can you see other ways to reduce unnecessary stress in your life?

Common Stress Solutions

There are some simple though indirect strategies for reducing stress:

• Improve your sleep habits.
• Exercise as tolerated regularly.
• Avoid chemical exposures.
• Eat balanced meals.
• Avoid people who are negative.

Stressor	Example	Rate	Possible Solution
1. Family stressors			
2. Social stressors			
3. Workplace stressors			
4. Environmental stressors			
5. Chemical stressors			
6. Financial stressors			
7. Physical stressors			
8. Emotional stressors			
9. Lifestyle challenges			

- Have a thankful attitude.
- Seek support from family, friends, and health-care providers.
- Don't take your job home with you.
- Learn to set boundaries by expressing your needs and saying "no" to those things or people who are toxic in your life.
- Make changing your lifestyle a priority.
- Ask yourself: "How important is this really? Will it make a difference one year from now?"

Grieving Your Losses

Studies have shown that chronically ill patients undergo a fairly predictable emotional response as they grieve for the loss of their health, their jobs, their income, and their self-esteem. To cope with this emotional duress, you may need counseling. It helps if this grief work can be done in a group setting so that you realize that when you have fibromyalgia or other chronic illnesses you are not alone and that others are having similar problems as a result of dealing with a chronic physical illness.

Emotional Stages of Grief in Chronic Illness

Denial
Conscious or unconscious refusal to accept facts, information, or the reality that you have fibromyalgia and as a result cannot work, for example

▼

Anger
Feelings of rage and envy over getting fibromyalgia

▼

Bargaining
The negotiation for an improved life is made with a higher power in exchange for a reformed lifestyle

▼

Depression
I'm so sad, why bother with anything?

▼

Acceptance
Individuals begin to come to terms with their fibromyalgia or chronic illness

The Challenge of Change

Managing your fibromyalgia involves making positive lifestyle changes to improve symptoms.

But making these changes is not always easy. Considerable research has been directed to the study of how we make changes in our lifestyle. There will be days when you "stay on track" and other days when you feel that you have "fallen off the wagon." Don't despair.

Yesterday is history
Tomorrow is
a mystery
Today is a gift
That's why it's
called the Present.

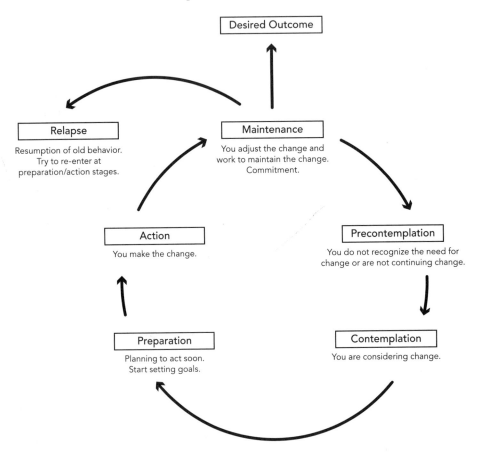

Adapted by permission from S Ekserci, *The Complete Weight-Loss Surgery Guide and Diet Program*, Toronto, ON: Robert Rose Inc, 2011.

Stages of Change

In their well-known "Stages of Change" model of behavior, James Prochaska and Carlos DiClemente describe five stages that a person goes through when wanting to change a behavior.

People embarking on change stay at different stages for various amounts of time. The process of change is ongoing. Having a strong support network to help maintain the lifestyle changes you have made is important.

Stage	Characteristics
Pre-contemplation	"Ignorance is bliss" Not considering change
Contemplation	"Sitting on the fence" Ambivalent about change Weighing the pros and cons of change Not going to make change in the next month
Preparation	"Testing the water" Planning to act within the next month
Action	Practicing new behavior for 3 to 6 months
Maintenance	Commitment to sustained behavior Post 6 months to 5 years
Relapse	"Fall from grace" Resumption of old behavior

Setting SMART Goals

Setting goals will assist you in achieving lifestyle changes. Like the Stages of Change model, the SMART model for setting goals will help you in the long run.

Specific

You need to be specific about what you want to accomplish. Focus on what you want to do.

Example: I maintain a slow and steady pace even on those days when I feel more energetic. I don't want to crash again.

Measurable

How will you measure your progress? How will you know you reached your goal?

Example: Every day I will fill in my activity log and compare it with logs from last week to see if I've improved my functional quality of life.

Achievable

Your goal should be attainable. Keep in mind your resources and ability. Is your goal achievable?

Example: I will be sure to go to bed before 10:00 p.m. and rise about 7:30 a.m. to reinforce my circadian rhythms.

Realistic

Is this goal attainable in your specified time frame?

Example: Yes, because I have taken my schedule into account.

Timely

Set up a time frame and a deadline.

Example: I will improve my diet and use the menu plans and recipes provided in this book, starting with shopping on the weekend and trying new breakfast menus on Monday.

Support for Change

Fibromyalgia can be a very lonely and isolating condition. You will need the support of those around you to understand the important changes you are making in order to heal. Friends may not understand that you can't make plans in advance as you often find yourself having to cancel based on how you are feeling. Family may not understand that you are not able to do all the chores around the house that you once could. Employers may not understand the accommodations necessary for you to heal. Unfortunately, many of your health-care workers may not

Q *What can I do to help my supporters help me?*

A Try these strategies. They are so self-evident that they are often overlooked.

- Educate your family, friends, and health-care providers about fibromyalgia.
- Try not to isolate yourself from those around you who can offer constructive support. Socialization is important (the parameters around your socialization may have to be modified).
- Ensure workplace accommodations are made.
- Ensure insurance forms are properly filled out.
- Ensure self-care strategies are in place, such as home care to give a bath and utilizing disability parking stickers if appropriate.
- Recognize the strength and beauty of who you are outside of accomplishments.
- Reframe your symptoms as early warning devices (e.g., increasing pain as your body communicating with you that it needs to rest and not that it is working against you).
- Celebrate your improvements, acknowledge your disappointments.
- Allow yourself to grieve the life you led. You need time to grieve your losses: your health, possibly your job, your lifestyle, and sometimes your family and friends.
- Seek out cognitive behavioral therapy or some other type of supportive counseling to help with the anxiety you may be experiencing and provide you with concrete stress management tools.
- Self-development: allow time for yourself; learn to trust your inner feelings and experiences.
- No longer push mind over matter. Allow your body to be supported and have a voice.
- Learn to set emotional and personal boundaries.

even understand. In fact, it is likely that you yourself are your hardest critic.

Self-Support

Remember — you cannot give someone else a glass of water unless your own glass is full. If an airplane is in an emergency situation, it is obvious that you need to put your own oxygen mask on before putting it on anyone else. It is not so obvious in life that you put your own mask on first in order to heal. The first person you need to ask support from is yourself. We have written a letter at the front of the book to help you educate your family and friends of your condition and what is needed to allow you to heal. It may also be helpful to find a support group with others who understand what you are going through. You may want to bring a close family member or friend to appointments so that they can better understand what you are going through and offer support.

Adaptation

The goal of lifestyle changes is to move from exhaustion to adaptation so as to achieve homeostasis or a balanced lifestyle. Effective lifestyle management strategies can transform stressors into the seeds of good health.

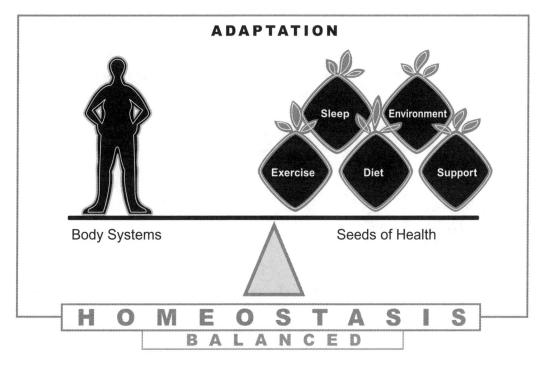

Adapted by pemission of Dr. Lynn Marshall, Environmental Health Clinic at Women's College Hospital, Toronto, Ontario.

CHAPTER 5

Medications for Fibromyalgia

Case Study

Anxious

Marion, who is 55, has had difficulty sleeping ever since she developed fibromyalgia. She became anxious because she was not sleeping well and her sleep worsened. She was taking a sleeping pill that was helping her get to sleep, but then she would wake up in the middle of the night feeling very anxious that she wasn't sleeping well and it would ruin the next day. After a while, she even began having trouble getting to sleep. She went to a support group for fibromyalgia, where she was taught about the sleep disturbances that were found in fibromyalgia. She also learned that getting anxious only made things worse.

In the class, Marion also learned about meditation and visualization. She started to practice meditation during her small rest periods throughout the day to help herself relax for a few minutes at a time. She started using meditation at night before she went to sleep, after she took her sleeping pill. She noticed that she found it easier to initiate sleep the nights that she meditated. Next she tried meditation when she woke up in the middle of the night and found that she could control her anxiety in this way. Even though she still had interrupted sleep, she felt better in the morning and had a better day when she meditated throughout the night.

Did You Know?

Muscle Relaxants

Some patients report that muscle relaxants — over-the-counter or prescription — help their muscles to relax and that they sleep better at night.

Although lifestyle changes can promote healing from fibromyalgia, at times something more may be needed. Sleep and pain medications, as well as antidepressants and anti-anxiety drugs, may be required to bear the symptoms of this syndrome.

Sleep Medications

Because you have fibromyalgia, you also have a sleep disorder. That's right. Sleep studies show conclusively that there is something physically and functionally wrong with your brain when you sleep. Drugs have been developed that can counteract this functional problem and enable you to sleep better.

Effective Sleep Medications

Before taking any medication, over-the-counter or prescribed, be sure to discuss with your pharmacist the recommended dosage and possible side effects. Do not change the dosage on your own without meeting with your physician. These medications have proven to be effective in managing sleep for patients with fibromyalgia.

- Dimenhydrinate (Gravol)
- Zopiclone (Imovane)
- Trazodone (Desyrel)
- Clonazepam (Klonopin, Rivotril)
- Doxepin (Aponal)
- Cyclobenzaprine (Flexeril)
- Mirtazapine (Remeron)
- Bromazepam (Lectopam)

Q *What do you recommend as the best sleeping pill?*

A There is no one particular drug that works better than the others. The one that works for you is the best medication for you. Follow the prescription dose and do not go beyond what is written on the prescription bottle. It is best if you keep the individual dose in a separate night time pillbox in case you wake up and don't remember if you took your pill. If the pill is not in the slot, you know you have taken it. This is one more safety precaution to help you to prevent accidentally taking too many medications at one time. You can buy pillboxes at the drug store, and some boxes even have morning, noon, dinner, and bedtime compartments.

Antidepressants and Anti-Anxiety Medications

If you are depressed or anxious as a result of dealing with your chronic illness, antidepressants or anti-anxiety medications can be helpful. The key is to find the one that works best in your body. Again, the rule of thumb is to start with a low dose and increase slowly until the medication is effective. The treatment of depression or anxiety with a chronic illness, such as fibromyalgia, is the same as the treatment of depression or anxiety without a chronic illness.

Sleep Management

Many of the anxiolytic medications (drugs that relieve anxiety) and antidepressants listed here have been found to be helpful in improving sleep quality in fibromyalgia. You at least feel as if you have had some sleep because your brain has been

Did You Know?

Controlled Dosage

If you require a sleep medication, start with a small dose. Some patients start with one-quarter of the normal recommended dose. If that dose helps initiate sleep, stay at that dose. If that dose doesn't help, increase the dose until the medication is effective, up to the recommended dosage.

Tired and Wired (Again)

Before taking any medications, first refer to the sleep section (page 39) and be conscious of your activity pacing. If you go to bed after you have pushed yourself to get "stuff" done all day, you are going to bed while you are crashing. Your body is exhausted but your brain is wired because it is on an adrenaline rush. We call this "tired and wired." Guess what? On these nights, your sleeping pill will not work.

unaware of your surroundings for a few hours. Unfortunately, none of the medications actually give you the deep sleep that is missing from your sleep cycle in fibromyalgia. Rather, they help improve your feeling that you did actually sleep. If your fibromyalgia symptoms, particularly pain, are improved then your sleep improves.

Pain Medications

Because you have fibromyalgia, you have pain all over your body: burning, stabbing, creepy-crawly pain. Pain that's light to the touch. If you feel intense pain when someone touches you, this is called hyperalgesia. In research studies, this symptom of fibromyalgia has been documented on functional MRIs (magnetic resonance images), which show an increased reaction to normal non-painful stimulation on the body. This condition is really tough emotionally when you can't stand your kids' hugs because they just hurt too much.

Managing Your Pain

How you manage your day will directly affect your ability to manage your pain. Does this sound familiar? To repeat: pacing is the number one concept that most impacts your pain. If you

Q *What is neuroplasticity?*

A Neuroplasticity refers to the brain's ability to adapt its structural and functional organization as a result of its experience. In other words, the brain learns how to interpret signals it receives on an ongoing basis and it changes how it functions as a result of these signals. In fibromyalgia, this means that too many neurons or brain cells are recruited abnormally in the interpretation of the fibromyalgia patient's pain signals. It is now thought that fibromyalgia pain is a central pain processing problem and that there is something physically and functionally changed within your brain. In other words, your brain is working overtime interpreting pain signals.

Unfortunately, functional MRIs are still research tools at this time. Documented abnormalities in fibromyalgia also include changes in single-photon emission computed tomography (SPECT) scans of the brain, increased levels of substance P in the cerebrospinal fluid, and decreased inhibition of pain pathways that help to reduce the sensation of pain. Substance P is a chemical in your body that is increased when you have chronic pain. The good news is that your brain can unlearn this abnormal functioning over time and — with techniques such as meditation and visualization — turn down the pain signal.

have pushed yourself to get "stuff" done all day, you are going to crash. Your body is exhausted but your brain is wired because it is on an adrenaline rush and your pain is much worse. We call this tired and wired. Guess what? On these days, your pain medication will not work very well because it is like giving an aspirin to a patient who has just come out of surgery — the pain is just too great. Is the solution to this problem to take more medication every time you crash? No! The key is learning how to pace yourself and to stop crashing so that your body has a chance to heal.

Coping with Pain

How do you go from a pain-centered life and break free from the pain spiral?

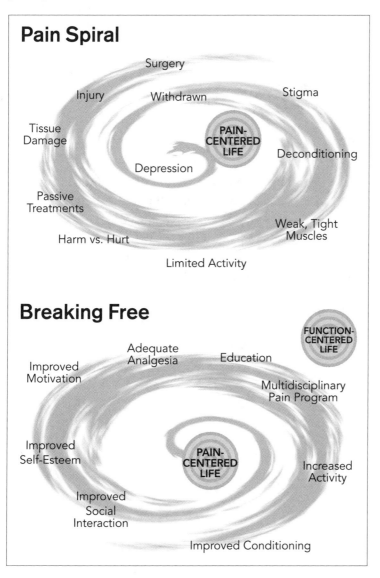

Pain Spiral

Surgery
Injury   Withdrawn   Stigma
Tissue Damage   PAIN-CENTERED LIFE   Deconditioning
Depression
Passive Treatments   Weak, Tight Muscles
Harm vs. Hurt
Limited Activity

Breaking Free

FUNCTION-CENTERED LIFE
Adequate Analgesia   Education
Improved Motivation   Multidisciplinary Pain Program
Improved Self-Esteem   PAIN-CENTERED LIFE   Increased Activity
Improved Social Interaction
Improved Conditioning

Regulated Pain Medication

The same rules apply for pain medication as for sleep medication. If you do require a pain medication, the rule of thumb is to start with a small dose. Some patients start with one-quarter of the normal recommended dose and — if needed — increase the dose to where the medication is effective.

The use of pain medications in fibromyalgia is not an exact science. Physicians will work with patients to determine if a medication works best for them. Pain medication is not a cure; rather, it is a supportive treatment used to reduce pain symptoms so that you can begin to move and have a more normal quality of life. A wide range of drug classes may help the pain.

Types of Pain Relief Medications

Some medications that are normally not thought of as pain medications have been found to be helpful in reducing the pain of fibromyalgia.

- *Anti-inflammatories:* Aspirin, Advil, Tylenol
- *Anticonvulsants:* pregabalin (Lyrica), gabapentin (Neurontin)
- *Tricyclic antidepressants:* amitriptyline (Tryptomer, Triplent), nortriptyline (Aventyl)
- *Selective serotonin reuptake inhibitors (SSRIs):* citalopram (Celexa), escitalopram (Lexapro), fluoxetine (Prozac, Sarafem), paroxetine (Paxil), sertraline (Zoloft)
- *Non-selective reuptake inhibitors (NSRIs):* venlafaxine (Effexor), milnacipran (Savella), duloxetine (Cymbalta), dopamine agonists
- *Opioids:* tramadol (Ultram, Ralivia)
- *Muscle relaxants:* cyclobenzaprine (Flexeril)

Pharmacologic Therapy in Fibromyalgia

A wide array of medications is prescribed for fibromyalgia symptoms, some with more scientific evidence supporting their effectiveness than others. All medications must be monitored for their effectiveness and possible side effects.

Evidence	Drug
Strong Evidence	Tricyclic antidepressant: amitriptyline (Tryptomer)
	Muscle relaxant: cyclobenzaprine (Flexeril)
	Dual reuptake inhibitors: serotonin-norepinephrine reuptake inhibitors (SNRIs) and the non-selective reuptake inhibitors (NSRIs) milnacipran* (Savella), duloxetine* (Cymbalta), venlafaxine (Effexor)
	Anticonvulsants: pregabalin* (Lyrica) and gabapentin (Neurontin)
Modest Evidence	Opiod: tramadol (Ultram)
	Selective serotonin reuptake inhibitors (SSRIs): citalopram (Celexa), escitalopram (Lexapro), fluoxetine (Prozac, Sarafem), paroxetine (Paxil), sertraline (Zoloft)
	Dopamine agonists: ropinirole (Requip), pramipexole (Mirapex)
	Gamma-hydroxybutyrate (Xyrem)
Weak Evidence	Growth hormone
	S-adenosyl-L-methionine (SAMe)

*Approved by the US Food and Drug Administration for treatment in fibromyalgia

Adapted from Goldenberg DL, et al. JAMA. 2004;292:2388–95.

Opioids

If your pain is moderate to severe, you may be prescribed opioids, beginning with a weak opioid, such as Tramadol. This should be reserved for treatment of patients with moderate to severe pain that is not responsive to other treatment modalities. Patients who continue to use opioids should show improved pain and function on their activity logs.

Your doctors will closely monitor you if you are taking opioids (which are narcotics) and will likely ask you to sign a contract while you are taking them. Your doctor will be looking for side effects, especially any signs of addiction, such as your early request for a prescription repeat of the pain medication or taking increased amounts of medication beyond the prescribed medication amount. Patients with severe pain can be monitored using random drug screenings of their urine to ensure that they are not taking any street drugs for their pain. Very complex and severe FM pain may require expert care under the supervision of a pain specialist.

Dextromethorphan

Dextromethorphan is another medication that has been prescribed for fibromyalgia pain. However, in our experience, it is best to avoid it. Dextromethorphan acts as a central nervous system stimulant. In other words, it overtaxes your brain — and then you push yourself too hard and crash. This is the exact opposite of the yin-building approach we have suggested in this book. You may experience a momentary boost when taking dextromethorphan, but it is not worth the fall and crash that may come after.

CHAPTER 6

Complementary Therapies and Alternative Medicines

Case Study

Abdominal Care

Joanna, a 53-year-old woman suffering from fibromyalgia, had been experiencing chronic constipation, causing abdominal discomfort and bloating. She noticed that her pain increased when she was constipated and was unable to eliminate waste. We prescribed a series of 6 weekly constitutional hydrotherapy sessions and probiotics. She agreed to increase her water intake to 8 glasses per day, and we recommended dietary changes consistent with the fibromyalgia nutritional plan outlined in this book.

After a couple of weeks, Joanna noticed she was having bowel movements every other day. By the end of the 6-week treatment, she was regular. She also noticed circulation side benefits following the hydrotherapy session (her feet were less cold and she felt slightly better able to adapt to fluctuations in temperature). In addition, her energy levels were higher than before starting the treatments.

Fibromyalgia is a chronic and systemic condition. This means that it can affect many different systems in your body, including, but not limited to, your brain (brain fog), your digestive tract, your urinary tract, your nervous system, your hormonal system, your musculoskeletal system, and your immune system. Trying to address each system with a treatment is not easy. However, complementary therapies and alternative medicines encompass many modalities of practice, from bodywork and hydrotherapy to nutritional supplements and Eastern (traditional Chinese) medicine.

Bodywork Therapies

Because fibromyalgia affects the musculoskeletal system (bones, muscles, tendons, and ligaments), it makes sense that bodywork therapies will be helpful in managing symptoms.

Massage Therapy

The physical manipulation of soft tissue can be extremely beneficial to patients suffering from fibromyalgia. Studies have shown a reduction in pain and anxiety, and improvements in sleep, mood, and energy levels, following regular massages. Substance P levels and a number of positive tender points have also been shown to decrease following massage.

Acupuncture

A traditional Chinese medicine treatment modality, acupuncture involves the insertion of very thin needles into specific points along the 12 meridian channels of the body. Acupuncture works to remove blockages along these channels. (In Eastern medicine, a blockage generates stagnation, which manifests as pain.) Acupuncture can be done both locally, by needling directly into areas of pain (called Ashi points), and constitutionally, by rebalancing yin and yang in the entire body.

There have been numerous studies showing the efficacy of acupuncture in decreasing pain, improving sleep, and improving mood. It can also be very helpful for a range of other health concerns, including digestive issues, headaches, and anxiety. The Mayo Clinic in the United States published a landmark study in June 2006 showing the efficacy of using acupuncture to improve fatigue, anxiety, and mood — with effects lasting up to 7 months following treatment. A nice benefit of acupuncture, and one of the reasons it is so effective with FM, is that all your symptoms are taken into account and are addressed in your treatment (rather than addressing them as separate entities). A recent study also showed promising results using cupping, which is essentially the act of dragging suction cups along meridians to break up stagnations, to reduce pain in patients suffering from fibromyalgia.

Craniosacral Therapy

Craniosacral therapy (CST) involves using gentle manual therapy to palpate and enhance the craniosacral system (membranes, tissues, fluids, and bones surrounding or associated with the brain and spinal cord) and to treat functional imbalances. The accessible areas of the craniosacral system include the cranial bones, the sacrum, and the coccyx. Craniosacral therapy has been shown to be effective at reducing pain in patients suffering from fibromyalgia. One study showed a significant reduction in pain at 13 of the 18 tender points following a 20-week course of craniosacral treatments. The results were still present 1 year following the treatment.

Osteopathic Medicine

Osteopathic manipulation is based on the functionality of the body's systems. Osteopaths work with soft and hard tissue, performing subtle manipulations that allow the body to regain balance and functionality. Studies have shown that osteopathic medicine improves functionality in patients suffering from fibromyalgia. One study showed that osteopathic medicine combined with standard conventional medical care was more efficacious in treating the pain associated with fibromyalgia than utilizing conventional medicine alone.

Hydrotherapy

Hydrotherapy is the therapeutic use of water to help manage pain relief. This modality includes contrast showers, cold-water treading, the application of alternating hot/cold treatments, and baths. Hot and cold each have healing properties. Caution: hot-water treatments are not advisable in patients with acute inflammatory conditions.

The Effects of Hot and Cold Water

Hot Water

- Dilates small blood vessels, increases blood flow, raises body temperature, and stimulates the healing process
- Helps to eliminate toxins through perspiration
- Relaxes muscles
- Relieves pain

Cold Water

- Reduces inflammation and constricts local blood vessels
- Stimulates the digestive system and the nervous system, improves muscle strength, and invigorates the body
- Reduces constipation and improves bowel function
- Increases energy and reduces fatigue
- Relieves pain

Contrast Shower

Contrast between hot and cold water increases circulation throughout your tissues, which in turn promotes detoxification, decreases inflammation, facilitates thermoregulation, and reduces fatigue. Contrast showers help your system rid itself of metabolic waste and inflammatory by-products. They have also been shown to increase the number of white blood cells and thus strengthen the immune system.

Did You Know?

Epsom Salts Baths

Some clinical research shows that balneotherapy (the practice of bathing to treat illness and injury) with mineral baths significantly reduces tender points in patients with fibromyalgia compared to baseline or no treatment. We recommend using 2 to 3 cups (500 to 750 mL) of Epsom salts in the bath in the evening to reduce pain and aid in sleep. It is important to ensure you are well hydrated and to ask for support if you have any problems getting in and out of the bathtub. If you experience any dizziness or lightheadedness, discontinue.

How to take a contrast shower

This type of shower involves 3 cycles of hot water followed by cold water. If you need to modify this program, ensure you at least finish your shower with cold water.

❶ Start with 3 minutes of hot water.
❷ Follow with 45 seconds of cold water.
❸ Repeat steps 1 and 2 two more times, making sure to end on cold water.
❹ Take a towel and dry off using a gentle friction rub.

You will likely not enjoy this the first couple of times you do it, but if you persevere, you will find that you start to crave the cold water at the end. You will also notice you are better able to regulate body temperature during the day and that you finish your showers feeling more energized and with less pain.

Cold-Water Treading

For those days when a shower is not possible or requires too much energy, cold-water treading is a great alternative to taking a contrast shower.

❶ Fill up the bathtub or a large bucket to the base of your calves and march in place. If needed, sit on the edge of the tub and swirl your feet.
❷ Do this in the morning for a maximum of 5 minutes.

Functional Medicine

Functional medicine is a proprietary process that refers to taking a whole-systems approach based on your individual biochemistry, genetic make-up, and individual needs. By doing the appropriate functional testing and assessing where imbalances are occurring on a cellular level, we can get closer to the root of the problem and provide objective measures. Although testing can be costly up front, it can end up saving money in the long term by streamlining supplements and interventions so that you only pay for what is individually relevant and necessary based on your intake and results. It can provide objectivity and direction in complex chronic cases, such as fibromyalgia. In essence, "functional medicine" refers to patient-centered care and to treating you as an individual and not as your condition.

Mind-Body Medicine

Acknowledging and harmonizing the connection between the mind and the body is essential to healing. The mind and body are inseparable — recent research has shown us that our thoughts can change our biochemistry. In times of stress, a common coping strategy is to compartmentalize the mind and body and try to separate them. The common pattern of mind over matter (or mind over body) then develops. It is vital that this disconnect be broken and that the body regain its voice. It is also vitally important that we understand and work with our thought processes such that we encourage constructive, positive thoughts that will have a positive influence on our overall health.

Deep Breathing

Taking very slow, deep belly breaths is one of the best ways to move from a sympathetic (fight or flight) state into a parasympathetic (rest and digest) state. A parasympathetic state is conducive to healing and encourages a reduction in adrenal overstimulation. In a proper deep breath, your abdomen should extend further than your ribcage. One strategy to incorporate deep breathing into your day is to schedule it at the start of all your meals. Taking a few deep breaths before eating will shift your system into a state that is conducive to eating (rest and digest) and will encourage mindfulness around eating.

How to use deep-breathing therapy

If you have never done it before, try this routine.

❶ Breathe in for a count of 4 seconds, hold for a count of 4 seconds, and breathe out for a count of 4 seconds.
❷ If counting to 4 is too much for you, try counting to 3.
❸ When you do deep-breathing therapy, you are not only relaxing your body, you are also relaxing your brain. Why? Because you cannot think and count at the same time.

Checking In

There is often a disconnect between our mind and body. This can be a source of anxiety and the result of years of placing mind over body. One useful exercise is to check in with your body throughout the day, asking yourself, "Body, in this moment, what do I need?" It doesn't need to be complicated. Just let your body inform you of its basic needs, needs that have likely been overlooked in the busyness of your life for years.

Harmonizing

There are several strategies and therapies to support the process of harmonizing mind and body, which in turn elicit the relaxation response.

Your body may ask you to:

• Eat	• Laugh	• Sleep
• Urinate	• Cry	• Rest
• Hug	• Drink some	• Stretch
• Breathe deeply	water	• Move

The first step is to let your body know you have heard its request. The next step is to honor your body's need. If you need to go to the bathroom, go to the bathroom. If you need to drink, have some water. If you need to rest, put your feet up and close your eyes — even if you don't have long. The important part is to acknowledge and honor your body to the best of your ability given the situation you are in. Typically there is a tendency to ignore the body and not pay attention until pain and fatigue well up.

Guided Imagery

Guided imagery is a useful tool for providing focus and direction to meditation. Guided imagery provides a script and story for the imagination to follow, eliciting the relaxation response and a profound sense of healing. There are some that are specific to conditions and symptoms, and ones that are more general, such as imagery based on a favorite place. Guided imagery can be a useful tool to quiet the mind before bed and aid in improving sleep.

Medical Bullying

No form of therapy should be used to try to "convince you" that you are not sick. This is a form of bullying or brainwashing that tries to change your belief system. The thinking is, if the therapist can change your belief system, you will be cured. Because fibromyalgia is not a belief system but a physical illness, this kind of bullying does not work. It is harmful to patients' self-esteem, and often they are pushed until they crash. I have seen patients crashed in bed for months afterward.

If you feel that you are not being listened to, that you are being asked to ignore all your body symptoms, and you are starting to crash as a result of the therapy you are in, tell your doctor what is happening so it is documented in your chart. You need to stop this harmful process immediately.

CHAPTER 7

Dietary Strategies for Managing Fibromyalgia

Case Study

Therapy Cocktails

Mary, a 45-year-old suffering from fibromyalgia, was experiencing many digestive concerns, including irritable bowel syndrome (IBS). We were concerned she was not able to digest and absorb the nutrients at the levels she needed from her foods and we prescribed a series of 6 Myers' Therapy Cocktails — the colloquial name for a nutrient mix (magnesium, calcium, and vitamins) that is administered intravenously. She noticed very little change after the first couple of treatments. She reported she felt more tired immediately after and always had to go directly home to lie down. After the third treatment, Mary still felt the increased fatigue immediately afterward, but noticed on her activity logs that her functional capacity level was higher during the rest of the week than it had been in previous weeks. We encouraged her not to push herself even though she was experiencing an increase in her energy level, and we emphasized the need to continue pacing herself. Mary continued to improve slowly but steadily over the course of the next 3 weeks. At the end of the 6 weeks, Mary moved to a monthly maintenance schedule. We also worked on healing and improving her digestive health to enable her to digest and absorb more of her nutrients through foods.

Fibromyalgia can be triggered by and treated with nutrients. Deficiencies of specific nutrients can leave the body prone to attack. Supplementing specific nutrients can counteract the onset of fibromyalgia symptoms. Discovering what nutrients are needed in the prevention and treatment of fibromyalgia is not an exact science, however. To introduce too many substances at once can have the opposite effect than the one you are hoping for. For this reason, approach nutritional therapy methodically and always consult with a health-care professional. Do not ingest products to treat specific symptoms; instead, take those that will help address the underlying causes of those symptoms.

Disclaimer

The actions, cautions, side effects, and dosage information on the nutraceutical and botanical medicines discussed in this book are based on current evidence-based research as cited in the references section of this book.

Nutritional Supplements

The nutrients listed here are rated according to the body of evidence proving their effectiveness. Recently, research in the field of nutritional therapy, also known as clinical nutrition, has grown exponentially. The information supplied here is as current and reliable as possible, so you can tailor your treatment plan with confidence. Part of healing is connecting your mind and your body. If you try a product and do not feel well on it, listen to this important information and consult with your health-care provider.

Fibromyalgia-Friendly Nutrients

- SAMe
- Coenzyme Q10
- Magnesium and malic acid
- 5 hydroxy-tryptophan
- D-ribose
- Probiotics
- Essential fatty acids (omega-3 and omega-6)
- Amino acids
  - Leucine
  - Isoleucine
  - Valine
  - Alanine
  - Glutamine
  - Glycine
- Melatonin

SAMe

Also known as S-adenosylmethionine, SAMe is a naturally occurring molecule found throughout the body, and it has been studied for the treatment of fibromyalgia. By acting as a methyl donor in many reactions in the body, it plays an important role in the biochemical reactions involved with hormones, neurotransmitters, proteins, and nucleic acids. It is found in decreasing concentrations in the body as we age. SAMe supplementation can be helpful for improving mood and sleep (it is associated with increased serotonin turnover and elevated dopamine and norepinephrine levels). SAMe can also be helpful for reducing pain and inflammation. As well, SAMe supplementation has been shown to increase the synthesis of glutathione, which plays an important role in the body's ability to detoxify.

Dosage: Studies have shown that a daily intake of 600 to 800 mg of SAMe can significantly improve the symptoms of fibromyalgia, such as mood and pain, as compared to placebo. Although taking supplements orally may be helpful, administering SAMe intravenously does not seem to reduce the symptoms of fibromyalgia as effectively.

Possible side effects and interactions: SAMe can cause gastrointestinal irritation and nausea. SAMe does have the potential to interact with some medications and natural substances that also act as antidepressants. Make sure to take SAMe only in consultation with your health-care provider.

Coenzyme Q10

Coenzyme Q10 (CoQ10) is a fat-soluble antioxidant that is important in the production of adenosine triphosphate (ATP), your body's primary energy source. CoQ10 is produced by the body. It is found in almost all cells, with a particular affinity for the heart (cardioprotective), kidney, pancreas, and liver. CoQ10 is also found in meat and seafood food sources, but not in high enough amounts to approach therapeutic doses. The primary use in the treatment of fibromyalgia is as an antioxidant, to counter the additional oxidative stress you are under and to help address the fatigue on a cellular level, thereby improving your functional capacity.

Dosage: One study looked at the combined effects of taking 200 mg of CoQ10 with *Ginkgo biloba* orally. This combination improved the patients' quality of life, taking into account improvements in overall health, physical fitness levels, emotional wellbeing, social activities, and pain.

Possible side effects: CoQ10 is typically very well tolerated. Rarely, CoQ10 can cause some gastrointestinal upset. Taking CoQ10 in divided doses minimizes the chances of any gastrointestinal side effects.

Magnesium and Malic Acid

In addition to its many other health benefits, magnesium itself is useful in the treatment of fibromyalgia because it reduces symptoms of muscle cramping and pain (both skeletal and smooth muscle), reduces migraine headaches, improves sleep, reduces anxiety, relieves constipation (in fact, the main side effect of taking too much magnesium is loose stool or diarrhea), and reduces fatigue (magnesium is concentrated in the mitochondria of the cells, where energy is produced). From a dietary perspective, magnesium is typically well absorbed from foods that are high in fiber. Dietary sources of magnesium are listed in the Food Sources of Fibromyalgia-Friendly Nutrients (page 98).

Did You Know?

CoQ10 Improvement

A recent study published in *Clinical Biochemistry* showed an altered distribution of CoQ10 in FM patients. The study suggests that the mitochondrial dysfunction and increased oxidative stress seen in FM patients is due to a defect in how CoQ10 is metabolized and utilized in FM patients. A follow-up study by the same primary author showed improvement in symptoms from supplementing with CoQ10 and further supports the use of CoQ10 with FM patients.

Pain Reduction

A study published in the *Journal of Rheumatology* suggests that malic acid combined with magnesium is safe and beneficial in the treatment of FM. It found significant reductions in the severity of pain and suggests remaining on the treatment for a minimum of 2 months.

Dosage: Our patients typically see a particularly effective reduction in fibromylagia-related pain and tenderness when magnesium is taken orally as a supplement in conjunction with malic acid (an alpha hydroxy acid). Studies also support this observation, showing that taking magnesium hydroxide plus malic acid orally seems to decrease fibromyalgia-related pain and tenderness. If supplementing without the guidance of a health-care provider, take 350 mg of oral magnesium as a maximum starting amount.

Possible side effects: Taking too much oral magnesium will cause osmotic diarrhea, so make sure not to ingest more than the maximum dose when starting.

5 Hydroxy-Tryptophan

Also known as 5-HTP, this product of the amino acid L-tryptophan is converted to serotonin in the body. Serotonin is important in regulating mood, appetite, sleep, and cognitive function (memory and learning).

Dosage: Taking 100 mg three times daily of 5-HTP orally appears to improve symptoms of fibromyalgia, including pain, stiffness, sleeplessness, and migraine headaches.

Possible side effects and interactions: 5-HTP can cause gastrointestinal upset. 5-HTP has the potential to interact with SAMe. Do not take if you are on antidepressants (SSRIs) or monoamine oxidase inhibitors (MAOIs).

D-Ribose

D-ribose is a five-carbon sugar found in the body. It is a critical molecule in the resynthesis of adenosine triphosphate (ATP), and thus extremely important in recovery from fibromyalgia.

Dosage: A pilot study published in the *Journal of Alternative and Complementary Medicine* concluded that taking a ribose supplement at a dose of 5 g three times daily increased energy and sleep quality, led to an improved sense of well-being, and decreased pain in patients with fibromyalgia. In terms of what we see in clinical practice, reviews are mixed. For some patients, we see a marked improvement, and for others, there's no change with supplementation. It seems most helpful for those who struggle to recover after physical exertion.

Possible side effects and interactions: D-ribose has the potential to cause gastrointestinal upset with symptoms such as nausea and diarrhea. Other potential side effects are headaches and low blood sugar.

Probiotics

Probiotics are live "friendly" bacteria that can be taken orally to recolonize the gastrointestinal tract and to take up real estate that harmful bacteria would otherwise occupy. In other words, they help to keep the problematic bacteria at bay. We commonly see a dysbiosis (bacterial imbalance) in the digestive tracts of our fibromyalgia patients. Healing the digestive tract is an extremely important part of treatment. More than 75% of your immune system resides in your digestive tract. The digestive tract has also been called your body's second nervous system based on the important role it plays in your nervous system. Because only a small amount of probiotics are found in yogurt, oral supplementation is needed to attain therapeutic levels.

Amino Acids

Finding the right balance of amino acids can be very helpful in the successful management and treatment of fibromyalgia. There are tests available through various laboratories in North America that measure levels of amino acids in the blood, and these can be done to develop an individualized treatment. Amino acids are the building blocks to proteins. They are also the building blocks of your neurotransmitters.

Branched-chain amino acids are essential amino acids (meaning that your body can't make these amino acids itself and they need to be consumed from dietary protein). Orally, branched-chain amino acids can be taken to prevent fatigue and improve cognitive function.

- Leucine
- Isoleucine
- Valine

Non-essential amino acids are amino acids that the body can make from other amino acids.

- Alanine
- Glutamine
- Glycine

Did You Know?

Myers' Cocktail

Administering intravenous nutrients allows them to enter the body without passing through the digestive tract. This can be extremely useful in cases where there are absorption issues. Intravenous therapy also allows for higher levels of absorption than would normally occur via the digestive tract. The standard Myers' Cocktail contains magnesium, calcium, vitamin B_{12}, vitamin B_6, vitamin B_5, B-complex, and vitamin C. Typically, patients report a reduction in pain and an improvement in overall energy and sense of well-being after receiving a treatment. We usually administer a series of 6 weekly infusions. It can take up to 3 treatments for some patients to notice an improvement, depending on how deficient and depleted they are.

Glycine acts as an anxiolytic, and studies have shown it may improve memory.

Melatonin

Melatonin is a hormone made by your pineal gland (tryptophan → 5-HTP → serotonin → N-acetylserotonin → melatonin). Melatonin's primary job is to regulate your body's circadian rhythm (and therefore your sleep patterns) and your body's endocrine secretions (hormones). Darkness stimulates the secretion of melatonin (light inhibits it) and this is why it is so important for you to sleep in a dark room and to not work or play on a computer before bed. Patients with sleep disorders related to fibromyalgia typically have low levels of melatonin. Studies have shown that melatonin may also decrease the severity and degree of pain in people with fibromyalgia.

Dosage: The typical dosing to improve sleep is 5 mg in the evening.

Possible side effects: Some patients report vivid dreams and nightmares after taking melatonin. In women going through menopause, melatonin has been associated with a renewal of their menstrual flow or light spotting. You should not drive or use heavy machinery for at least 5 hours after taking melatonin.

Food Sources of Fibromyalgia-Friendly Nutrients

Deficiencies in these nutrients can trigger fibromyalgia. Be sure to eat foods rich in these nutrients to manage your illness.

Nutrient	Food Source
Vitamins	
Vitamin B$_1$	Sunflower seeds, legumes, nuts
Vitamin B$_2$	Legumes, spinach, leafy green vegetables, nuts
Vitamin B$_3$	Fish, dandelion greens
Vitamin B$_5$	Sunflower seeds, avocado, cooked salmon, baked winter squash, saltwater fish, nuts, legumes
Vitamin B$_6$	Chicken, fish, peas, spinach, legumes, sunflower seeds, avocado
Vitamin B$_{12}$	Legumes, nuts, fish, lamb

Nutrient	Food Source
Vitamin D	Halibut, salmon (Exposure to sunlight and full-spectrum light also causes the body to manufacture vitamin D)
Minerals	
Calcium	Sesame seeds, cooked turnip greens, cooked spinach, lamb's-quarters, sardines with bones, cooked collard greens
Copper	Sunflower seeds, sesame seeds, dried beans, Brazil nuts, walnuts, cashews, peas, quinoa
Iodine	Sea salt, sea vegetables (edible seaweeds), cod, garlic, onions, fish
Iron (heme)	Red meat (heme iron), blackstrap molasses, cooked amaranth, fortified cereals (gluten-free), pumpkin and squash seed kernels, white beans, beets, asparagus, nettle tea, lentils, sardines, leafy green vegetables (e.g., Swiss chard)
Magnesium	Legumes (black-eyed peas), vegetables (Swiss chard, avocado, broccoli, squash), nuts and seeds (pumpkin, cashews, especially almonds), whole grains (brown rice), fish
Omega-3 fatty acids	Eicosapentaenoic acid (EPA) and docosahexaenoic acid (DHA): oily ocean fish are the best source (sardines, anchovies, salmon, mackerel) Alpha-linolenic acid (ALA): flax seeds, hemp, walnuts, dark green leafy vegetables
Potassium	Swiss chard, avocado, cooked pumpkin
Selenium	Brazil nuts, baked halibut and snapper, Swiss chard, seaweed
Amino Acids	
Arginine	Almonds, nuts, seeds, turkey, chicken, lamb
Carnitine	Beef, fish, chicken
Glutamine	Wild game, turkey, chicken
Lysine	Turkey, halibut, salmon
Methionine	Salmon, wild game
Tryptophan	Turkey, lamb, cashews, avocado, halibut, salmon, wild game
Tyrosine	Wild game, turkey, spirulina

Botanical Medicine

Traditionally, medicinal plants have been used to treat symptoms of diseases and syndromes like fibromyalgia. Recent research has shown that certain plants are in fact therapeutic for fibromyalgia. Although we can reduce botanicals to their biochemical constituents in order to understand their mechanism of action in our bodies, there is much more to a plant than this. Many plants work well in combination with other plants, drugs, and nutrients, but it is important that you consult your medical practitioner and only combine these substances under supervision. Please note that some of these botanicals interact with sleep and other medications.

Pain Management
Turmeric

Turmeric is a natural anti-inflammatory. It has been found to be comparable to ibuprofen in its ability to reduce pain in patients suffering from other inflammatory conditions, such as osteoarthritis and fibromyalgia.

Dosage: The dosage range is 500 mg twice daily to 500 mg four times daily.

Capsicum

Capsicum applied topically (externally) can be helpful in decreasing pain. The mechanism for this effect is thought to be that the topical application of capsicum causes substance P to be released. Substance P is a sensory neurotransmitter that mediates pain. Repeated applications of capsicum are thought to result in substance P depletion, causing a desensitization and subsequent reduction in pain.

Dosage: The topical application of a capsicum cream (containing 0.025% of the active capsicum constituent capsaicin) four times daily to tender points for 4 weeks has been found to reduce tenderness in patients with fibromyalgia.

Adaptogens

Adaptogens are substances that help you adapt to stressors in your environment. The adrenal glands, as part of the hypothalamus-pituitary-adrenal axis, have been overtaxed in the case of fibromyalgia. Certain herbs have been shown to be effective in reversing this condition. Clinically we have seen the value of supporting our fibromyalgia patients with adaptogens. Be sure you are using non-stimulating support (avoid *Panax ginseng*, for example) or it may provide you with a sense of transient energy and will ultimately be feeding your yang while masking your yin deficiency — and thus eventually lead to an even greater fall.

Withania somnifera (Ashwaghanda)

Ashwaghanda is used as an adaptogen and general tonic. It can be a helpful component in the treatment of insomnia and anxiety and has also been found to improve cognitive function and decrease inflammation. In addition, it has immunomodulating effects. If you are having arthritic-like pains, you may also find an added benefit to taking this herb (it is used in the treatment of arthritis). It can be taken as a tea or tincture, or in capsule form.

Dosage: The dosage range is 1 to 6 g daily as a capsule or as a tea.

Rhodiola rosea (Golden root)

Rhodiola is an herb that can increase energy, strength, and endurance. In fibromyalgia, rhodiola can be beneficial in improving cognitive function, thereby helping with the symptoms of brain fog. It can also be helpful in supporting your body in times of stress (yin building) because it acts as an adaptogen for adrenal support, helping the body better adapt to stressors.

Dosage: For improving fatigue, *Rhodiola rosea* can be taken at 340 mg twice daily (3% rosavin, 1% salidroside).

Sleep Herbs

Several herbs are well known as sleep aids with few or no known side effects.

Valeriana officinalis

Valerian is a useful herb in the treatment of insomnia and sleeping disorders. It can also be helpful in patients whose sleep worsens with the hormonal changes associated with menopause.

Dosage: The oral dosage is 400 to 900 mg of valerian extract in the evening. It can also be used topically by adding it to your bathwater to decrease anxiety and promote a more restful sleep. Valerian can combine well with lemon balm (*Melissa officinalis*) to improve sleep. For some patients, valerian seems to have

Did You Know?

Like Cures Like

Homeopathy works under the premise of like cures like. Vaccines are an example of like cures like, by exposing the body to a foreign antigen to evoke an immune response, which prepares the body for a larger, subsequent exposure. Homeopathics are very dilute substances. They are so dilute in fact that there is often no measurable amount of active constituent in them. The more dilute, the less matter and thus the stronger it is from an energetic perspective. Because homeopathics work on a different level than botanical medicines, they are safe with other medications.

the opposite effect intended and can contribute to excitability, insomnia, and vivid dreams.

Passiflora incarnata (Passionflower)

Passionflower is used for insomnia and can settle the digestive tract if stress has caused gastrointestinal upset. It can also be helpful in treating symptoms of opiate withdrawal. Passionflower makes a nice evening tea to help promote better-quality sleep.

Dosage: Passionflower can be taken as a tea 30 minutes before bed by mixing 0.25 to 2 g in ⅔ cup (150 mL) of hot water and steeping the mixture for 15 minutes, then straining.

Homeopathic Remedies

Homeopathy remains a controversial area in medicine. It is an energetic medicine, meaning it works on a different level than most medicines. It is also an individualized form of medicine in which your health needs to be considered in its entirety — mind, body, and spirit — in order to select the correct remedy and truly heal.

Homeopathic Remedies for Fibromyalgia

Arnica for trauma; bruised sensation
Hypericum for shooting/radiating nerve pain
Gelsemium for a feeling that you are too weak to sustain the pain; weak and/or dizzy and want to lie down; feel paralyzed from the pain
Rhus toxicodendron (Rhus Tox) for pain worse after periods of rest; arthritic-like pains
Complex homeopathics such as Neurexan for aid in sleep
Ignatia for a sense of loss/grief
Complex homeopathics such as Nervoheel/Rescue Remedy for treating anxiety

Did You Know?

Homeopathic Testing

A placebo-controlled crossover study published in *Rheumatology* demonstrated that individualized homeopathic prescribing is significantly better than placebo at improving global health and quality of life and reducing pain in FM patients.

CHAPTER 8

Eastern Medicine Protocol

Case History

Eastern Paradigm

Recently, Helena was diagnosed with fibromyalgia. Prior to becoming ill, Helena had always been very high functioning. She was a single mother of two children and she worked shift-work as a nurse. However, years of poor sleep and poor eating habits had left her in a survival state, run down and exhausted. From an Eastern medical perspective, she was in a very yin deficient state relative to her yang energy.

About a year ago, Helena was in a car accident and felt a sharp decline in her health. From an Eastern perspective, her yang declined following the accident. She had already been in a very deficient state. When her false energy plummeted, Helena found herself pathologically fatigued, with full body pain and severe brain fog. This can be explained by the yang's sharp decline, leaving Helena with a relative excess of yin (which is still very deficient, but is now higher than yang).

Yin is slow and chronic in nature. Yin is water. Helena was now in a stagnated (or stuck) damp pattern (brain fog, pain, symptoms worse in damp weather). She tried to push through by self-medicating, drinking coffee and taking other stimulants to make it through the day. She soon noticed that she had entered into a crash cycle.

Occasionally, she would have days she felt better. Yang is acute in nature with a short wavelength and high amplitude. In other words, yang can come up quickly but will not last without the substance from yin to balance it. In these periods when she felt better, she would try to go back to her old ways to accomplish as much as she could and try to recover some of the life she was grieving the loss of. Not surprisingly, she found herself feeling worse than before she relapsed. From an Eastern medicine perspective, in these times she pushed too hard, she had further depleted her yin and burnt more of her yang energy, thus falling even further than before.

The treatment in this case was to help Helen rebuild yin. For every activity on the yang side, an extra deposit must be made into the yin side. We can think of yang as activity and yin as rest. We approached treatment from a yin-building perspective. This approach takes patience and time, but it is necessary to get out of the crash cycle and begin to heal. Yin support means supporting the parasympathetic system through proper sleep, rest, pacing, and eating habits. "Does this build or deplete me?" For every answer that is "deplete me," an extra deposit on the build side (or yin side) must be made.

Eastern medicine offers an alternative approach to or a paradigm for healing fibromyalgia that focuses on the balancing of yin and yang energy in the body.

Balanced Yin and Yang Energy

When you are healthy, there is a balance of yin and yang energy in your body. Yin and yang should ideally co-exist in a dynamic equilibrium. They are interdependent and one cannot exist without the other.

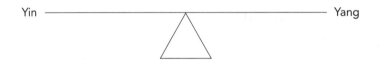

Yin Energy Depletion

Fibromyalgia is a condition that causes you to be extremely depleted physically. Long before your fibromyalgia began, your yin energy was likely depleted, the result of years of stress, poor sleep, overwork, poor diet, trauma, genetic predisposition, and hormonal changes. For the most part, your yin was depleted by your hectic lifestyle. This depletion of yin energy left you with a relative excess of yang. Think of yin as your rest and digest state and yang as your fight or flight state. When you are in this depleted yin state, you are in a continuous fight or flight, adrenalin-charged state. When you are pushing yourself to do more than you should do, you are tapping into your sympathetic nervous system to get you through the day. In this state, you rely on false energy, such as coffee or sugar, to give you a quick but false energy fix. In this state, you are "running on empty," tapping into your adrenal glands for a quick fix of adrenalin to keep on pushing yourself to get stuff done. Some patients are actually adrenalin junkies and don't remember what normal energy feels like. They are continuously in a state of "go go go," with the mind ignoring the body.

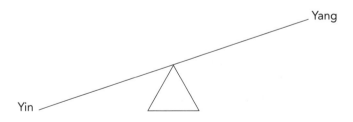

Total Energy Depletion

If, while in a state of depleted yin energy, you experience a physical trauma that causes your yang energy to drop sharply, you will find yourself deficient in both yin and yang, though there will be a relative excess of yin — slow and damp — manifesting as brain fog, pain, and fatigue.

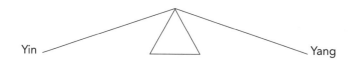

Rebuilding Protocols

Rebuilding your health means supporting the yin energy as well as rebuilding the yang energy in the body so that the body goes back into a balanced energy state. It is tempting to focus on rebuilding yang and neglecting yin, as yang is to yin as energy is to matter. In other words, you can feed into the yang by adding stimulating therapies that will give an energy boost, which may be very tempting. Yang is much quicker to come back, but as it

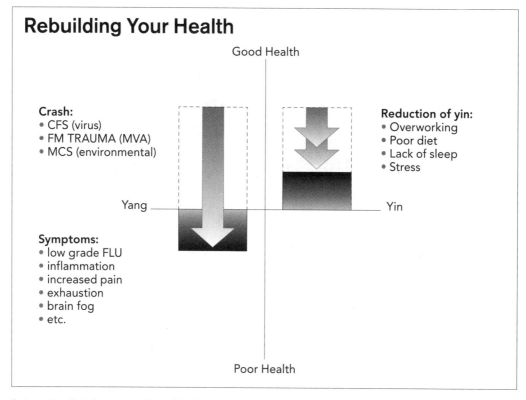

Eastern medicine illustrations courtesy of Louise S. McCrindle and Alison C. Bested.

While fibromyalgia cannot be "cured" with a single silver bullet, many people with fibromyalgia are able to improve their quality of life and, in some milder cases, experience recovery by rebuilding their yin and yang.

also has a much shorter wavelength, it will be quick to fall back down (and each time lower than the first) if it is not supported by yin. It is essential you follow the tortoise and the hare model and rebuild yin. Slow and steady restorative yin-building therapies will prevent the big crashes that occur as a result of feeding the yang and neglecting the yin. In terms of pacing, yang can be considered activity while yin can be considered rest.

Rebuilding Yin

You have likely not felt well since you experienced a trauma while in a state of depleted yin. Now you are experiencing fatigue (yin is slow), increased pain (yin is damp stagnation), and you have brain fog (a cloud of yin). Rebuilding your health means supporting your yin energy and yang energy so that the body goes back to a balanced energy state.

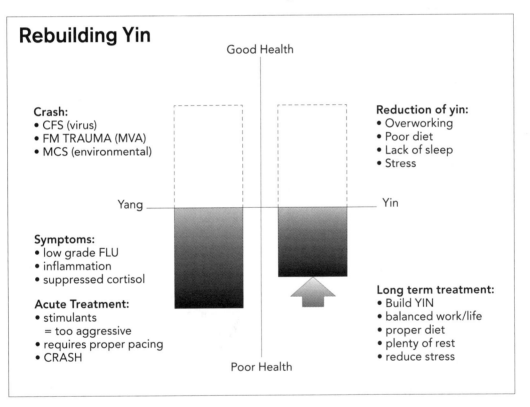

Rebuilding Yin

Good Health

Crash:
• CFS (virus)
• FM TRAUMA (MVA)
• MCS (environmental)

Yang

Symptoms:
• low grade FLU
• inflammation
• suppressed cortisol

Acute Treatment:
• stimulants
  = too aggressive
• requires proper pacing
• CRASH

Reduction of yin:
• Overworking
• Poor diet
• Lack of sleep
• Stress

Yin

Long term treatment:
• Build YIN
• balanced work/life
• proper diet
• plenty of rest
• reduce stress

Poor Health

Rebuilding Yang

It is tempting to focus on rebuilding yang energy and to neglect yin energy. You can feed yang by adding stimulating therapies that will give you an energy boost.

Yang is quick to rebound because it has a much shorter wavelength, but it will be quick to fall back down (and it will fall lower than the first fall) if it is not supported by yin strategies.

Slow and steady restorative yin-building therapies will prevent the big crashes that occur when yin is neglected.

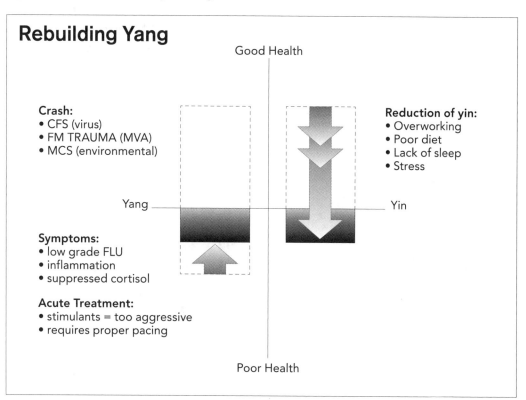

Rebuilding Yang

Good Health

Crash:
• CFS (virus)
• FM TRAUMA (MVA)
• MCS (environmental)

Reduction of yin:
• Overworking
• Poor diet
• Lack of sleep
• Stress

Yang —   — Yin

Symptoms:
• low grade FLU
• inflammation
• suppressed cortisol

Acute Treatment:
• stimulants = too aggressive
• requires proper pacing

Poor Health

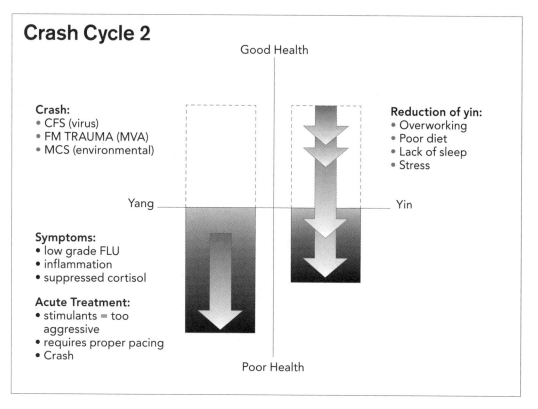

Crash Cycle 2

Good Health

Crash:
• CFS (virus)
• FM TRAUMA (MVA)
• MCS (environmental)

Reduction of yin:
• Overworking
• Poor diet
• Lack of sleep
• Stress

Yang —   — Yin

Symptoms:
• low grade FLU
• inflammation
• suppressed cortisol

Acute Treatment:
• stimulants = too aggressive
• requires proper pacing
• Crash

Poor Health

Pacing Yourself

In order to heal, you must rebuild your yin by ensuring better sleep, improving your nutrition, pacing yourself — and being good to yourself. Here is where the SEEDS management program and Eastern medicine merge. It will be tempting as your yin rebuilds to go back to your old ways, but remember how disagreeable life was when your fibromyalgia was in full swing. Balancing yin and yang is a lifelong exercise.

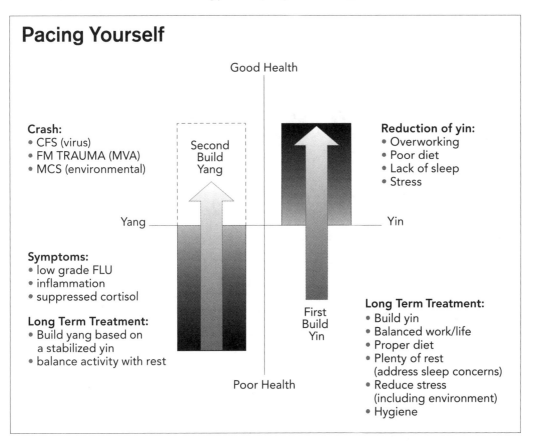

Pacing Yourself

Good Health

Crash:
- CFS (virus)
- FM TRAUMA (MVA)
- MCS (environmental)

Second Build Yang

Reduction of yin:
- Overworking
- Poor diet
- Lack of sleep
- Stress

Yang

Yin

Symptoms:
- low grade FLU
- inflammation
- suppressed cortisol

Long Term Treatment:
- Build yang based on a stabilized yin
- balance activity with rest

First Build Yin

Long Term Treatment:
- Build yin
- Balanced work/life
- Proper diet
- Plenty of rest (address sleep concerns)
- Reduce stress (including environment)
- Hygiene

Poor Health

Part 3

Fibromyalgia Diet Program

CHAPTER 9
Dietary Therapy

Case Study

Mindful Eating

Jacqueline, a 58-year-old woman with fibromyalgia, came to see us and complained of extreme brain fog, pain, and fatigue. She was working as a producer at a national television station, a very challenging environment with long hours and high demands. In the past, she had been able to push through, but she was finding it increasingly difficult to accomplish what she once could. This was very frustrating to her because she was used to being a high performer in her job.

At our first visit, we spent some time discussing diet. Jacqueline felt that overall she was eating quite well. We gave her a simple diet diary she could use to chart exactly what she was eating over the course of the week. Putting the information on paper forced her to look at her diet as a whole, rather than as a series of meals, and — like many of our patients — she was quite surprised to see what she was actually eating.

Because Jacqueline had been having great difficulty sleeping through the night, she was often not able to get out of bed until midday on her days off. This meant that her first meal was around noon and she was missing breakfast completely. She also realized she was consuming much more sugar than she initially thought, particularly in the late afternoon when she was at her lowest and needed a quick pick-me-up.

We decided to have Jacqueline try our fibromyalgia diet program, which focuses on avoiding pro-inflammatory foods and enjoying anti-inflammatory foods. This diet is designed to reduce overall inflammation in the body. Inflammation results in excess swelling, redness, heat, and pain. By changing the foods in her diet, we were able to reduce Jacqueline's overall body inflammation at the cellular level and thereby help reduce her fibromyalgia pain. She was resistant at first when she looked over the food list, worrying about it being too restrictive and feeling overwhelmed at the thought of making all the changes. We decided to approach it by working on one meal at a time until all of her meals and snacks worked within the program guidelines. We tackled breakfast first — ensuring that she was eating breakfast every day and that it followed the recommendations. Once she felt confident with her options for breakfast meals, we moved on to lunch and so forth.

Jacqueline followed the program guidelines strictly for 3 weeks. Like many of our patients, she reported that the first week was the most challenging. She was irritable and frustrated by not being able to eat her typical go-to foods. We encouraged her to continue, and by the time she was in week 2, she reported a significant decrease in pain, an improvement in energy and sleep quality, and a decrease in brain fog. By the time she had finished the full 3 weeks, she did not want to reintroduce, or challenge, any of the foods she had so reluctantly taken out, for fear that her symptoms would return to their previous state.

However, we did encourage her to challenge these foods and methodically reintroduce them in an effort to identify her specific food intolerances, and to allow her to reintroduce those foods that, although a common allergen, may not be an allergen for her. The reintroduction phase also allowed her to eat in a more mindful way — experiencing how the different foods specifically affected her. Jacqueline reintroduced each food methodically, one at a time, and found that tomatoes increased her pain; that dairy foods resulted in gastrointestinal issues, such as bloating and discomfort, as well as increased fatigue; and that gluten increased pain, brain fog, and fatigue. Jacqueline decided to remove these foods from her diet and continues to improve. She also reports a side benefit: she has lost 20 lbs (9 kg) while enjoying new foods and meal ideas, which got her out of her old food rut.

Perhaps the single most important therapy you can implement is to return to the basics and look at what you are eating. Some foods will sooth your fibromyalgia symptoms, others will aggravate them. Knowing the foods you can enjoy and the foods you should avoid is not that difficult if you follow these guidelines.

Fibromyalgia Diet Program
Balanced
High protein
Omega-3 rich
Low carbohydrate
Hypo-allergenic
Organic
Anti-inflammatory

Nutritional Status

Before you start changing your diet, work with your health-care professional to establish a nutritional baseline. This will give you a reference point to track your nutritional progress and reveal any nutritional deficiencies you may be experiencing. These deficiencies can trigger or aggravate fibromyalgia. They might even be a causal factor.

Special Nutrients

Some minerals and vitamins have a special role to play in recovering from fibromyalgia. Your doctor will likely test your blood for the presence of these minerals and vitamins. You can also have nutrients tested through hair and urine analysis, although these tests are a subject of debate over their accuracy.

Nutrient Deficiencies

If you are low in certain nutrients, it may be because you are lacking them in your diet or you are eating them but cannot digest, absorb, or retain them. In that case, you can have a stool analysis done to investigate your digestive functions.

Food Allergy

Other tests can be used to detect any food allergies, intolerances, and sensitivities you may have that are the result of your fibromyalgia or a trigger for symptoms.

Keep a 7-Day Diet Diary

Another way to evaluate your nutritional status is to keep a 7-day diet diary.

Instructions for completing a 7-day diet diary

❶ Using the accompanying tables, write down everything that passes your lips for 1 week. Record what you eat for breakfast, lunch, and dinner, plus any snacks in between. Be sure to record any beverages, including water, that you drink and the quantity. The more specific you can be, the better. For example, if you eat a sandwich, include the type of bread and all of the ingredients; don't just write "sandwich."

❷ Keep the diet diary with you and write everything down immediately after eating rather than trying to remember at the end of the day — or, even worse, at the end of the week!

7-Day Diet Diary Table

Day	Breakfast	Lunch	Dinner	Snacks	Symptoms
Day 1					
Day 2					
Day 3					
Day 4					
Day 5					
Day 6					
Day 7					

❸ Monitor what times you are eating and write the information down. Are you eating at regular times? Are you skipping meals?

❹ Note any symptoms you have while or after you eat. Do you have gas or bloating after eating certain foods? Is your pain worse? Is your brain fog worse? Is your sleep worse? The diet diary will help you become aware of what you are eating and how it is affecting you. You will see patterns of related foods, called food groups, and their effects on your body and emotions. If any meal or ingredient triggers or aggravates a symptom, make a note of this in the right column.

❺ Note how your body reacts to eating different types of foods. Track your symptoms to see if they improve with the dietary changes recommended in this book.

Q *How do you interpret the results of the diet diary?*

A Look at what you have eaten and compare it to the nutritional guidelines of the fibromyalgia diet program. We suggest using a few colored pencils or highlighters to help with the interpretation and to emphasize the observations you are making. Highlight any deviations from the program, but without judgment. Simply observe. Note any corresponding increase or decrease in symptoms and your overall sense of well-being. Because the severity of your symptoms likely fluctuates on a day-to-day basis, the key is to look for overall patterns. For example, whenever you eat tomatoes, you experience a migraine headache. Or perhaps on the days you have no sugar, your mood is more stable and you have a better night's sleep.

Do not view any deviations from the program as a failure, but rather as an opportunity to explore your obstacles and to problem solve around them in order to make realistic and long-term change. An example of this would be: you find yourself reaching for something sweet to eat at 9:00 p.m. This is a perfect opportunity to stop and be mindful — in other words, check in with yourself.

- Ask your body what it needs from you. If your answer is that you are tired, it means that you need to go to bed now and not half an hour from now.
- You may be using food as a source of quick energy, to push yourself to be able to do more and get a second wind at night. Try to avoid pushing yourself before bedtime because you will be tired physically but wired mentally and you'll be unable to sleep when you do actually go to bed.
- If the answer is that you are stressed, what do you need to do to reduce the stress? Try taking 10 deep abdominal belly breaths or doing a guided meditation. Chances are, you won't feel like eating the sweet afterward.
- Perhaps you are lonely or bored. What would help you fill this void? Try doing a gratitude journal or calling a friend or family member for a brief chat.

- Perhaps when you look back at your diet diary for the day, you realize you did not have enough protein and healthy fats and thus you are now hypoglycemic (your blood sugars are low). If this is the case, you may want to have a handful of raw almonds and highlight this on your diet diary to ensure you are focused on incorporating enough the following day. A diet diary can provide an amazing amount of insight into your health.

Micronutrients for Managing Fibromyalgia

If you are deficient in any one of these nutrients, your health may be compromised and your fibromyalgia symptoms may be aggravated. Standard blood tests will detect the level of most of these nutrients, though special tests may be needed for some.

Minerals

Calcium: essential for building and maintaining healthy bones, muscle function (leg cramping can be due to low calcium levels, for example), heart function, and release of neurotransmitters

Chloride: an essential electrolyte regulated by the kidneys; necessary for metabolism, nerve impulse transmission, and maintaining the body's proper pH (acid-base balance)

Chromium: an essential trace element important for blood sugar regulation

Cobalt: a key component of vitamin B_2

Iodine: essential for your thyroid's ability to produce thyroid hormone (which regulates metabolism)

Iron: forms complexes with hemoglobin, which function as oxygen-transport molecules in the body

Magnesium: many enzymes depend on magnesium to function (including those involved with ATP, your body's "energy currency"); important for proper calcium absorption; and important in proper muscle function and nerve transmission

Manganese: a cofactor for many important enzymatic reactions in the body

Molybdenum: essential for protein synthesis in the body, and essential to some enzymatic reactions in the body, including purine catabolism

Phosphorus: part of the building blocks of life (as a component of DNA and RNA) and a component of ATP (the body's "energy currency")

Potassium: an important electrolyte key to proper nerve transmission and maintaining the proper balance of fluid between and within cells

Selenium: important in the proper functioning of the thyroid gland and a component of some enzymes in the body, including glutathione peroxidase (antioxidant enzyme)

Sodium: an essential electrolyte vital to regulating blood pressure, fluid balance, and pH in the body

Zinc: essential for proper development and growth, immune function, and proper functioning of the central nervous system and brain

Vitamins

Vitamin A: necessary for vision (seeing in low light and in color) and proper immune function

B vitamins (B_1, B_2, B_3, B_5, B_6, B_{12}, choline): essential for proper cell metabolism (energy production, enzymatic reactions, growth, development, neurotransmitter synthesis, and nervous system health

Vitamin C: a common cofactor in numerous enzymatic reactions, essential for collagen formation (wound healing), acts as an antioxidant, and assists with iron absorption

Vitamin D: essential for absorption of phosphate and calcium in the gastrointestinal system, necessary for bone health, and important in the immune system

Vitamin E: important antioxidant and plays role in the immune system and numerous enzymatic reactions

Vitamin K: essential in blood clotting, bone metabolism, and good health

Amino Acids

Histidine: an important transport molecule, important for the absorption of calcium, blood-clotting effects, and decreases histamine levels in the body (and therefore has anti-inflammatory effects)

Isoleucine: required for the formation of hemoglobin, helps regulate blood sugar levels, and important in muscle recovery

Leucine: involved in wound healing; helps regulate blood sugar levels; involved in the growth and repair of bones, skin, and muscle

Lysine: involved in collagen formation (wound healing) important to the health of connective tissues in the body, essential for growth, involved in the production of carnitine (which is responsible to shuttling long-chain fatty acids through the mitochondria of cells to be used for energy), and has some antiviral effects

Methionine: involved in fat metabolism, acts as a strong antioxidant, important role in the immune system, and important for proper detoxification

Phenylalanine: important in the synthesis of neurotransmitters and therefore involved in mood regulation, memory, and learning

Threonine: important in collagen formation, important for proper liver functioning, plays role in mood support

Tryptophan: required to make the neurotransmitter serotonin, which is important for healthy brain function, including mood support, sleep regulation, and pain reduction

Valine: an important energy source for muscles; essential for proper muscle function, tissue growth, and repair

Essential Fatty Acids

Omega-3 fatty acids: have important anti-inflammatory effects, concentrated in the brain and important in cognitive and behavioral health, and important for normal growth and development

Omega-6 fatty acids: important for healthy brain function, growth, and development; can be pro-inflammatory if they are not in balance with omega-3 fatty acids

Probiotics: necessary for the production of the B vitamins in the intestines and necessary in maintaining healthy immunity of the intestinal lining

Food Basics

Our food can be broken down into two categories, macronutrients and micronutrients. Macronutrients include protein, fat, and carbohydrates. They provide us with the energy needed to live. Micronutrients enable the breakdown of macronutrients into energy. They include minerals, vitamins, amino acids, and essential fatty acids.

Proteins

Proteins are made up of one or more chains of amino acids. They are the building blocks of life. They directly and indirectly supply our body with significant energy and are necessary for the growth and repair of tissue, for the synthesis of enzymes in the body, for hormone and neurotransmitter synthesis, for detoxification, and for building antibodies to fight off infection.

High-Protein Diet

The fibromyalgia diet is a high-protein diet, rich in essential amino acids. A high-protein diet is important for improving energy levels, reducing pain, and improving mood, sleep, and cognitive function. It achieves this by helping to regulate blood sugars, thereby reducing ups and downs in energy levels, and by providing your body with the essential amino acids important for such things as the growth and repair of tissue, proper muscle functioning, your body's enzymatic reactions, your immune system, your endocrine system (hormones), and the synthesis of your neurotransmitters.

Fats

Fat is composed of fatty acids, or lipids. They are essential for maintaining a healthy weight and metabolism. They are also an important component of feeling satiated and thus prevent overeating.

There are three basic kinds of fat: saturated, unsaturated, and trans. Saturated and trans fats have been linked to a host of health concerns, but unsaturated fats (polyunsaturated and monounsaturated) are an important source of energy for the body and enable the absorption of fat-soluble vitamins (A, D, E, and K).

Essential fatty acids (EFAs) are so named because our bodies cannot produce them by themselves. They are important for regulating hormones, growth, mood support, immune function, and decreasing inflammation.

There are two forms of EFAs: omega-3 and omega-6 fatty acids. Omega-3 acids include alpha-linolenic acid (ALA), eicosapentaenoic acid (EPA), and docosahexaenoic acid (DHA). An ideal diet should have an omega-6 to omega-3 ratio of 2:1. In North America, the ratio is closer to 20:1. Research has shown that omega-3 fatty acids benefit a wide range of conditions, including fibromyalgia, depression, arthritis, cardiac arrhythmia, cancer, diabetes, mood disorders, and skin diseases.

Omega-3-Fatty-Acid–Rich Diet

The fibromyalgia diet is rich in omega-3 essential fatty acids, which help regulate hormones, mood, immune function, inflammation, and fibromyalgia symptoms.

Did You Know?

Complete Protein

Meat is the only complete source of protein. It contains all the essential amino acids that the body cannot make in sufficient quantities to support life. The exception is quinoa, which is a non-animal-based complete source of protein. Plant sources of protein include legumes, nuts, and seeds. You can still get all the essential amino acids in sufficient quantities through a vegetarian diet; however, you must be sure to combine your plant proteins in such a way that you are not missing any.

Carbohydrates

Carbohydrates are an organic compound consisting of carbon, hydrogen, and oxygen. They are the major source of energy in the diet. There are two types of carbohydrates: simple and complex. Simple carbohydrates are refined carbohydrates that contain simple sugars. The body uses up simple carbohydrates quickly, causing a rapid rise and fall in blood sugar. They are also highly refined and carry little nutritional value. Glucose-fructose syrup is used to sweeten drinks and baked goods. It is 55 times sweeter than table sugar. There are concerns that it is contributing to obesity, cardiovascular disease, diabetes, and non-alcoholic fatty liver disease. Complex carbohydrates are non-refined and promote good health by keeping blood sugar levels low.

Glycemic Index

Carbohydrates are categorized by their position on the glycemic index (GI), which measures how quickly the glucose from a particular food enters the bloodstream, and by glycemic load (GL), which measures the quantity of carbohydrates (sugars) in a particular food. Limit the high-glycemic carbohydrates in your diet to maintain a healthy weight and reduce the risk of diabetes and heart disease.

10 Common High-GI Foods to Avoid or Restrict

Food	GI	GL
1. Bagel	69	24
2. Bread, white	78	12
3. Dry toasted Os cereal	74	15
4. Raisins	64	28
5. French baguette	83	15
6. Pancakes, buckwheat, from mix	102	23
7. Honey	87	18
8. Potatoes, white, baked	98	26
9. Rice pasta, brown	92	35
10. Jasmine rice, white	109	46

10 Common Low-GI Foods to Enjoy

Food	GI	GL
1. Barley	22	9
2. Broccoli	0–15	1.5
3. Celery	0–15	1.5
4. Cherries	22	3
5. Chickpeas	36	11
6. Cucumber	0–15	1.5
7. Green leafy vegetables	0–15	1.5
8. Lentils	29	5.0
9. Onions	20	1.5
10. Zucchini	0–15	1.5

Example of Low-, Moderate-, and High-Glycemic Foods

Low-Glycemic Foods	Moderate-Glycemic Foods	High-Glycemic Foods
Broccoli	Black-eyed peas	Rice crackers
Leafy green vegetables	Buckwheat	Cookies
Legumes (chickpeas, soybeans, green peas, lentils)	Bulgur	White bread, bagels
Nuts	Sweet corn	Chips
Rice bran	Pasta, whole wheat	Cereal, sweetened
Cucumber	Mango	Soda, sweetened
Apples	Kiwi	Bananas
Pears	Orange	Ice cream
Cherries	Apple juice, unsweetened	Juices with added sugar
Berries	Sweet potato, yam	White potatoes, baked
Grapefruit	Pumpkin	Waffles, pancakes
Peach	Grapes	Dates, raisins
Barley	Brown rice	White rice

Glycemic Index and Load Guide to Food Groups

Vegetables	GI	GL
Alfalfa sprouts Bok choy Broccoli Brussel sprouts Cabbage Cauliflower Leafy green vegetables: chard, kale, mustard greens, Chinese cabbage, collard greens, dandelion, endive, escarole, lettuce, spinach, turnip greens, beet greens Parsley Watercress	0-15	1-2
Artichoke Asparagus Bean sprouts Celery Cucumber Fennel Okra Onions Radishes Rhubarb String beans (green or yellow) Summer squash Zucchini	0-20	1-2
Pumpkin	51	3
Sweet potatoes	48	16
Yams	54	19
Parsnips	52	4
Potatoes, baked	98	26
Potatoes, boiled	49	15
Carrots	33	2
Sweet corn on the cob	48	8
Sweet corn	55	9

Grains	G	GL
Rice bran, extruded	19	3
Barley	22	9
Millet	71	26
Bulgur	46	12
Brown rice	50	16
Arborio risotto rice	69	36
White basmati rice	52	24
Buckwheat	49	15
Instant rice	87	36
Tapioca, steamed	70	12
White jasmine rice	109	46

Beans (legumes)	GI	G
Soybeans	15	1
Green peas	22	2
Kidney beans	29	7
Lentils	29	5
Split yellow peas	32	6
Lima beans	32	10
Chickpeas	36	11
Black beans	30	7
Pinto beans	33	8
Black-eyed peas	52	16

Fruit	GI	GL
Cherries, raw	22	3
Peach	28	4
Apricots, dried	30	8
Kiwi	58	7
Orange	40	4
Watermelon	72	4
Pineapple	66	6
Apple	34	5
Grapes	49	9
Apple, dried	29	11
Prunes, pitted	29	10
Pear	33	4
Mango	51	8
Grapefruit	25	3
Banana	58	13
Raisins	64	28
Dates, dried	62	21

GI and GL values referenced from www.glycemicindex.com

Common Digestion Problems

If you have fibromyalgia, you are likely prone to digestive, absorption, and retention problems. These symptoms can include:

- Cramps
- Gas
- Bloating
- Diarrhea
- Constipation
- Acid reflux
- Other symptoms similar to those seen in irritable bowel syndrome (IBS)

Low-Carbohydrate Diet

The fibromyalgia diet is a low-carbohydrate diet, low in carbohydrate quantity, and low on the glycemic index. This component of the fibromyalgia diet increases your energy levels and reduces brain fog while helping to prevent fluctuations in blood sugars. In patients with fibromyalgia, we commonly see functional issues with the breakdown of carbohydrates (obstacles in the biochemical pathways necessary for effective utilization of carbohydrates). Minimize simple carbohydrates if there is an underlying issue with yeast or molds: simple carbohydrates are readily broken down into sugars, which yeast and molds thrive on.

Food Guides and Groups

To achieve basic good health in the face of fibromyalgia, we recommend following a modified anti-allergenic and anti-inflammatory version of the food guides created by the United States Department of Agriculture (USDA) and Health Canada. Both the USDA MyPlate program and Health Canada's Eating Well with Canada's Food Guide will help you eat a well-balanced diet that resolves most nutrient deficiencies and avoids food triggers.

Food Groups

Both the USDA and Health Canada categorize foods into groups and recommend the number of servings of these food groups that will maintain good health at different ages and stages of your life.

- Vegetables
- Fruit
- Grains
- Nuts and seeds
- Legumes and beans
- Meat and meat products
- Dairy and dairy products (and dairy alternatives)
- Condiments
- Sweeteners
- Beverages

How to Divide Your Plate

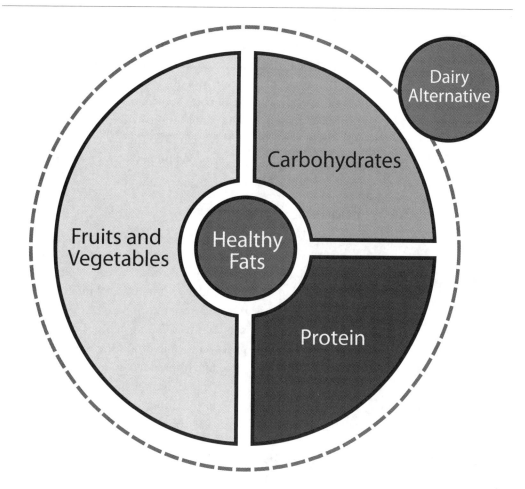

10 tips to a great plate

These are based on the USDA food guidelines, which we've modified to meet your specific dietary needs.

1. Balance calories.
2. Enjoy your food but eat less.
3. Avoid oversized portions.
4. Eat more vegetables, fruits, and gluten-free whole grains.
5. Make half your plate fruits and vegetables.
6. Switch to dairy-free alternatives.
7. Make half your grains whole grains.
8. Cut back on foods high in solid fats, added sugars, and salt.
9. Compare sodium in foods and select low-sodium or no-salt-added products.
10. Drink water instead of sugary drinks.

Food Allergies and Intolerances

The human immune system is designed to protect the body from potential harm. Allergies are an abnormal immune reaction. The substance that triggers an allergic response in people is called an allergen. Some people have abnormal immune responses to foods. We all know someone who is allergic to shrimp or peanuts. Some people are so extremely allergic that it is life-threatening — this means they have an anaphylactic response. Other people have food intolerances or sensitivities to the foods they eat.

Food Allergy

The body can react abnormally to food in a variety of ways. When you eat a food that you are allergic to, your body produces an immunoglobulin or antibody against the food. One of the immunoglobulins it can produce is immunoglobulin E (IgE). IgE causes cells to produce histamines. These histamines cause the common allergy symptoms, including itchiness, swelling, running nose, watery eyes, coughing, wheezing, shortness of breath, hives, rashes, and mucus production. It can even cause a severe reaction called anaphylaxis, one that is potentially fatal and includes the swelling of the throat and tongue. Allergic responses and the severity vary from person to person.

Food Intolerance

Some people lack specific digestive enzymes that help to digest food. For example, many adults do not have the digestive enzyme lactose, which helps to digest milk and dairy products. When they drink milk, they do not digest and absorb it. Instead, they get diarrhea from the undigested milk and milk products. These people are described as being deficient in lactose and can purchase milk that includes the digestive enzyme.

A food intolerance may have an immediate or a delayed response. These responses are thought to be a result of the body's release of cytokines as a response to the exposure to the specific food. A cytokine is a chemical protein molecule, one that has been more recently discovered in the immune-system response. Food-intolerance symptoms can include bloating, gas production, diarrhea, constipation, skin conditions (such as eczema), fatigue, and brain function problems, such as brain fog and difficulty thinking, remembering, and concentrating. Usually these reactions are not life-threatening.

Did You Know?

ELISA

The enzyme-linked immunosorbent assay (ELISA) is a common clinical test for food allergies. Your health-care professional can help you contact a lab that will conduct this test and help you read the results.

---

10 Most Common Food Allergies and Intolerances

- Peanuts
- Tree nuts (walnut, hickory)
- Seafood
- Milk
- Eggs
- Soy
- Wheat
- Sesame seeds
- Sulfites
- Mustard

Elimination Diet

To determine if you have a food allergy or intolerance to a specific food or food group, consider following an elimination, or challenge, diet strictly for 3 weeks.

1 Select one food or food group to be tested (for example, milk). Remove it from your diet for 3 weeks. Do you notice any improvement or aggravation of your fibromyalgia symptoms? In the case of milk and milk products, you will most likely respond favorably to their removal.

2 After 3 weeks, methodically reintroduce the food you excluded. Do you notice any return or aggravation of symptoms? In the case of milk and milk products, you will likely respond unfavorably.

3 If — after 3 days of consuming this reintroduced food — you notice no change in symptoms, move on to another food.

4 If you do notice a change, remove the food immediately, wait until symptoms dissipate, and then proceed to the next item on the list.

Hypo-Allergenic Diet

The fibromyalgia diet is hypo-allergenic, meaning it avoids or eliminates various foods that cause allergic reactions. Dairy foods are especially problematic for most people with fibromyalgia.

Organic Foods

Consume organic foods when possible. This will reduce your exposure to antibiotics, hormones, and potentially harmful irradiated food that can trigger or aggravate allergies and fibromyalgia. The foods you eat should be free of preservatives, artificial colors, and additives. Organic foods best meet this need for "clean" food.

Did You Know?

Processed and Fried Foods

White flour products, such as cookies, cakes, and pastries, should be avoided if you have fibromyalgia. Processed foods are likely to house harmful chemical ingredients, such as monosodium glutamate (MSG). There is also very little nutrient value in these foods, and they often contain trans fats and are often high in sugar. Because most fibromyalgia patients already have compromised digestive tracts that interfere with the proper absorption of nutrients, it is imperative the foods consumed provide ample nutrients.

Deprivation Diet

The typical Western diet is composed largely of pro-inflammatory foods, such as dairy, red meat, and nightshades (tomatoes). When reviewing the list of pro-inflammatory foods, you may be left wondering, "What is left for me to eat if I remove all of these?" Don't worry: this is far from a deprivation diet. In fact, you will be able to eat a wide variety of foods that better regulate your blood sugars, decrease inflammation, improve digestive health, and better meet all of your nutritional needs.

Top "Dirty" Foods

A "dirty" food is one that has been treated with pesticides. The Environmental Working Group in the United States has published a list of the most important "dirty" foods. Choose organic versions of these foods, even if they are slightly more expensive.

- Apples
- Celery
- Strawberries
- Peaches
- Spinach
- Nectarines (imported)
- Grapes (imported)
- Bell peppers
- Potatoes
- Blueberries
- Lettuce
- Kale
- Collard greens
- Fatty meats (e.g., pork fat)
- Milk
- Coffee
- Wine
- Chocolate

Top "Clean" Foods

The Environmental Working Group has also published a list of "clean" foods that are not heavily treated with pesticides. You can save money on these foods because they don't need to be organic.

- Onions
- Corn
- Pineapple
- Avocado
- Asparagus
- Peas, sweet
- Mango
- Eggplant
- Cantaloupe (domestic)
- Kiwifruit
- Cabbage
- Watermelon
- Sweet potatoes
- Grapefruit
- Mushrooms

Adapted by permission from the Environmental Working Group.

Inflammatory Foods

Clinically, we see that fibromyalgia symptoms can be lessened when inflammatory foods are eliminated from the diet. Although we lack scientific studies and research that is specific to these nutritional interventions and fibromyalgia, there are numerous studies showing that changing the diet can cause changes in blood markers for inflammation, such as C-reactive protein.

If inflammation is reduced, it follows that someone suffering from fibromyalgia will experience less pain and an improvement in quality of life, which is what we typically see with our patients.

Q *What is inflammation?*

A Inflammation is swelling, redness, heat, and pain produced in the body as a reaction to injury or infection. This can happen locally or throughout the whole body. The body is trying to protect itself from harmful threats, such as infection, injury, and foreign substances. It does this to rid itself of the problem and to heal.

In the acute phase of inflammation, for example right after an injury, common symptoms include redness, heat, and swelling. Acute inflammation is in fact an important part of healing.

Sometimes inflammation becomes chronic, and this is a problem because the reaction lasts longer than the body needs to heal, and tissue around the inflamed area begins to suffer as a result. This happens when the body does not turn off its inflammatory response. There are different types of chronic inflammation in the body. Some of the symptoms of chronic inflammation include chronic pain, fatigue, skin problems (such as chronic hives), and gastrointestinal issues (such as food allergies or intolerances).

Low-Inflammatory-Food Diet

The fibromyalgia diet program is free of the foods that are commonly known to cause inflammation in fibromyalgia patients.

Pro-Inflammatory Foods to Avoid

The fibromyalgia diet is an anti-inflammatory one. Pro-inflammatory foods should be avoided.

Vegetables to Avoid

- Some nightshade family vegetables (tomatoes, potatoes, eggplant, and bell peppers). Nightshade vegetables contain a chemical alkaloid called solanine, which triggers inflammation. Yams, sweet potatoes, and squash are allowed.
- Corn and corn products (including popcorn). These cause a rapid increase in blood sugar. Corn is also a common food intolerance and can therefore contribute to inflammation.
- Mushrooms. Mold can sometimes be present on mushrooms, which should be avoided in patients with fibromyalgia.

Fruits to Avoid

- Some citrus fruits. Oranges and grapefruit can be acid-forming and inflammatory. Please note that lemons are permitted because they are alkaline-forming in the body.
- Sulfured or sugar-coated dried fruits. Sulfur dioxide is used as a preservative in dried fruit. Many fibromyalgia patients

are sensitive to the preservative. The sugar-coated dried fruit spikes blood sugars. Dried fruit should also be avoided because it can contain mold.

- Grapes and grape skins. Grape skins can sometimes be moldy.

Grains to Avoid

- All gluten-containing grains (wheat, spelt, rye, oats, and barley). These are commonly found in breads, pasta, and other products prepared using refined flour. Gluten may lead to inflammation.

Q *What is gluten?*

A Gluten is a protein consisting of a mixture of glutelin and gliadin, present in cereal grains, especially wheat. These protein molecules are very large and hard to digest, especially in people with food sensitivities or absorption problems. Gluten may create a state of chronic, low-level inflammation throughout the digestive tract and other parts of the body, such as the brain, joints, and tissues. In susceptible individuals, a gluten-free diet is recommended to enhance overall health. For fibromyalgia patients, digestive problems, brain fog, and issues related to weight management may resolve or significantly improve when a gluten-free diet is closely followed.

Nuts and Seeds to Avoid

- Peanuts and peanut butter. Peanuts are a common food allergen and contain aflatoxin (a potentially carcinogenic mold).
- Pistachios.
- Nuts and seeds that are salted or flavored.
- Peanuts, pistachios, and nuts and seeds that are salted or flavored can all contribute to inflammation.

Legumes to Avoid

- Soybeans and soy products (tofu, soy milk, soy sauce, tempeh, and textured vegetable protein, or TVP). Soy is a common food intolerance, which can contribute to inflammation. From an Eastern medicine perspective, it is also damp-forming, which fibromyalgia patients want to avoid.

Fish to Avoid

- Seafood/shellfish. Seafood and shellfish are common allergens and have higher risk for elevated mercury levels.

- King mackerel, tilefish, swordfish, shark, and tuna steaks. These fish are often contaminated with mercury.

Meats to Avoid

- Red meat. Inflammatory studies have shown that red meat could contribute to an increased risk of cancerous tumors. Please note that the quality of meat is directly related to what the animal eats. (Livestock is commonly fed corn, but there are recent reports that claim some cattle are now being fed candy due to the increasing price of feed.)
- Pork. Pork is one of the most difficult foods to digest. Cured and preserved pork is high in nitrites (associated with many adverse health effects). There is also an increased parasite risk with pork.
- Canned meat and cold cuts. Canned meat and cold cuts are processed meats that have nitrites and nitrates, which are added to preserve and enhance flavor and color. There is a link with bladder cancer and these preservatives. These processed meats are often also high in sodium. Canned meats and cold cuts can also contribute to inflammation.

Dairy Foods to Avoid

- All dairy products — milk, cheese, yogurt, and eggs. These need to be avoided because dairy can trigger inflammation.

> **Q** *Why are dairy foods banned when I've been told they are essential for strong bones and teeth?*
>
> **A** Dairy is a common food intolerance, which can trigger inflammation (manifested as pain). Interestingly, from a traditional Chinese medicine perspective, fibromyalgia is considered a damp condition manifested as pain, brain fog, and fatigue. Dairy is an extremely damp-forming food. Goat milk and cheese tend to pose fewer food-intolerance problems than products derived from cow's milk.

Oils to Avoid

- Canola oil and other vegetable oils (sunflower, safflower, corn, soybean). Vegetable oils are extracted from seeds such as the rapeseed (canola oil), but they cannot be extracted naturally; instead, they are chemically removed and altered. Fibromyalgia patients do best with unaltered, clean foods. Note that margarine and shortening are derived from vegetable oil, which undergoes an additional process called hydrogenation (this is what makes it solid).

Sweeteners to Avoid

- Refined sugar (white or brown). Refined sugar causes large fluctuations in blood sugars, which fibromyalgia patients want to avoid. Refined sugar is also devoid of nutrients.
- Artificial sweeteners (NutraSweet and aspartame, for example). The less likely a substance is to be found in nature and the more we have altered it, the less likely it is that our bodies know what to do with it and it can thus become a harmful substance to ingest. There are animal studies linking aspartame to cancer, for example. Aspartame is also known to suppress the thyroid gland (this is ironic given all the "diet" drinks that contain it).
- High-fructose corn syrup. High-fructose corn syrup is usually found in processed foods. In addition to the sugar issue for fibromyalgia patients, there is evidence that the body has difficulty metabolizing high-fructose corn syrup. There are also links with high-fructose corn syrup and increasing rates of type 2 diabetes.

Q *Why are sweeteners and sugars so problematic if you have fibromyalgia?*

A Many people often crave foods containing sweeteners and sugars. The reason for this may be multifactorial: you are sleep-deprived and therefore the hormones you secrete in your sleep, such as leptin and ghrelin, which are responsible for regulating appetite and satiation, are out of balance. You are pathologically fatigued and feeling the need for a pick-me-up. You may have skipped one or more meals and may not have had enough fat and protein in the day to feel satiated. The reason sweeteners and sugars are so problematic is that eating them doesn't solve any of the underlying reasons you may be craving them. In fact, it compounds the problem and makes you feel even worse in the long term. If you are suffering from sleep dysfunction, having your blood sugars rise rapidly and then fall throughout the day will further interrupt sleep patterns at night. This rise and fall in blood sugars will only increase energy transiently and you will experience a sharp decline in energy soon after, making you feel even more fatigued than before. In addition, sweeteners and sugars tend to be devoid of nutrients and fill the space that nutritious foods could be occupying. As a result, your body will still be craving nutrients following your consumption of sugars and you will not feel satiated.

Beverages to Avoid

- Coffee, caffeinated beverages, energy drinks, and sodas. Because your adrenals are already in need of ample support, you want to stay away from stimulating substances, such as coffee (think of the yin/yang description — you want to build and nourish yourself, not inject false energy that causes your core to further deplete). If you feel you absolutely cannot function without coffee, make extra sure you are resting at night and pacing yourself, ensuring that you don't let the coffee mask your underlying need for rest and nourishment. Sodas are high in sugar and numerous other chemicals that you need to avoid (diet soda is even worse for added chemicals).

- Alcohol. Avoid drinking alcoholic drinks because they can sometimes contain mold.
- Vinegars (apple cider is an exception). Vinegars should be avoided because they can sometimes contain mold.
- Do not drink any liquids with your meals because this dilutes your stomach acids and makes it more difficult to properly digest your food.

Q *Are energy drinks safe?*

A Energy drinks are the worst of the worst beverages. They combine the negatives of caffeine with the negatives of high-fructose and high-sucrose beverages. Be wary of even those marketed as using natural extracts, because they are still made up of stimulants that will spike and crash your energy levels (and, in the short term, this may mask your need for rest). These stimulants are often addictive, both mentally and physically, and they become a crutch on which to function, even if at a low level. In the long term, they will prevent your healing because they are pushing your body in the exact opposite direction it needs to go in order to repair.

Anti-Inflammatory Foods

The fibromyalgia diet is an anti-inflammatory diet that avoids or eliminates specific foods that promote inflammation and includes foods that reduce inflammation. The following guidelines feature information on what the fibromyalgia diet program entails and how to best prepare these foods. The way you eat can be as important as what you eat. In these guidelines for preparing items in the various food groups, we have highlighted a list of anti-inflammatory foods to be enjoyed.

Did You Know?

Anti-Inflammatory Spices

If you have fibromyalgia, you can enjoy all kinds of spices, especially turmeric, which has potent anti-inflammatory properties.

Anti-Inflammatory Food List

In your effort to reduce your fibromyalgia symptoms and fully recover, select these foods to eat. How to prepare these foods is explained following this list of anti-inflammatory foods, and these foods are the key ingredients in the recipes at the back of this book.

Vegetables	• All fresh vegetables (except the nightshades, which are pro-inflammatory) • Onions, leeks • Garlic • Carrots • Beets • Celery • Cauliflower	• Brussels sprouts • Cabbage • Green beans • Broccoli • Asparagus • Sweet potatoes, yams • Leafy greens: kale, mustard greens, turnip greens, bok choy, kohlrabi
Fruit	• All fresh fruits (except bananas, citrus, and dried fruits that are pro-inflammatory)	• Fruit sauces • Baby foods with no added sugar
Grains	• Brown rice • Millet • Buckwheat • Quinoa	• Tapioca • Teff • Amaranth
Legumes	• All legumes (except soy, which is pro-inflammatory) • Adzuki, black, and navy beans	• All peas: fresh, split, and snap • Lentils (any variety)
Nuts and Seeds (Raw)	• Almonds, walnuts, cashews, Brazil nuts, pecans	• Sesame seeds, sunflower seeds, pumpkin seeds
Meats, Poultry, Fish	• Free-range chicken and turkey (or grain-fed if organic is not available) • Organic lamb	• Wild game • Wild deepwater fish: salmon, halibut, cod, mackerel, sardines
Oils	• Olive, sesame, flax	
Sweeteners	• Stevia, agave, honey, maple syrup	
Spices	• All herbs: parsley, coriander, garlic, ginger, basil	• All spices: ground curry, fennel seeds, cayenne pepper, ground cinnamon, ground cloves, sea salt
Sauces	• Spreads: tahini paste, nut butters (almond, hazelnut, sesame, sunflower, cashew), apple butter, bean dips (hummus)	• Sauces: pesto without additives, mustard without additives, apple cider, brown rice vinegar, freshly squeezed lemon juice

Anti-Inflammatory Food Preparation Guide

These dietary recommendations are excellent for reducing inflammation, which occurs in any condition where pain is involved and in all chronic degenerative diseases.

Vegetables

- Steam or bake your vegetables. This decreases the work your digestive system needs to do to absorb nutrients, allowing the gastrointestinal (GI) mucosa to repair itself. It is okay to use flash-frozen, precut vegetables, saving you time and energy.
- Consume minimal raw vegetables, except as salad or juiced. Juicing is best for poor digestion or digestive problems.
- Add your favorite herbs and spices to enhance the taste of these vegetables.
- Enjoy eating from the following list of vegetables: onions, garlic, carrots, beets, leeks, broccoli, leafy greens, sweet potatoes, squash, yams, Brussels sprouts, cauliflower, celery, cabbage, green beans, and asparagus.

Fruits

- Eat only 1 to 2 servings of fruit daily. Although fruit can be nutrient-rich, it is also a source of sugar, which is not favorable for those with fibromyalgia.

Grains

- Eat non-gluten grains, such as basmati or brown rice, rice crackers, millet, quinoa, amaranth, buckwheat, teff, tapioca, and arrowroot.

Nuts and Seeds

- Eat raw, unsalted nuts and seeds (for example, almonds, sunflower seeds, chia seeds, pumpkin seeds, and walnuts).
- Sprinkle or grind them over your cereal, cooked grains, or salads, or eat them as a snack. You may also enjoy nut and seed butter spreads (for example, raw almond butter).

Legumes and Beans

- Enjoy all dried beans, peas, and lentils. Legumes are full of nutrients (B vitamins, folate, calcium, and potassium) and are high in fiber. They help regulate blood sugars and are satiating.
- Dried beans and legumes should be rinsed and soaked overnight before cooking.

- You can prepare extra beans and legumes and freeze them for future meals by immersing cooked legumes in cold water, draining, and freezing.
- Although canned legumes and beans are not ideal from a nutritional standpoint alone, they are an option if cooking the legumes is too taxing and depleting (and a preferred option to overdoing it and crashing later).

Fish and Seafood
- Eat a variety of fish. Focus especially on eating fish high in omega-3 fatty acids (salmon, mackerel, anchovies, sardines, herring). Among its many benefits, omega-3 fatty acids help decrease inflammation and improve mood. Note that the average intake of omega-3 fatty acids in the United States is only 13% of the recommended 1000 mg daily (as recommended by the American Heart Association).
- Poach, bake, steam, or broil fish.
- Try to purchase wild or Pacific fish, rather than farmed or Atlantic fish, because they have lower levels of pesticides, organochlorines, polychlorinated biphenyls (PCBs), and dioxins.

Meat
- Eat only the white meat (no skin) of chicken and turkey. Free-range or organically grown poultry and beef is preferable because meats have been found to be contaminated with growth hormones, pesticides, and herbicides.
- Enjoy wild game and lamb, which tend to be leaner than domesticated animals.
- Bake, broil, or steam all meat. Avoid barbecuing or charring meat, specifically the fat on meat, because it can be carcinogenic.

Note that toxins tend to accumulate in the fatty portions of meat.

Dairy Foods
- Do not consume dairy products, though you can eat dairy substitutes, including rice milk, nut milk, and coconut milk (in moderation).

Oils and Butter
- Enjoy coconut oil, cold-pressed extra virgin olive oil, flaxseed oil, and fish oil.
- Never heat flaxseed oil or fish oil because heating damages these oils.

- Fish oil is best for decreasing inflammation. Use it generously (aim for 2 g daily).

Sweeteners

- Enjoy very small amounts of natural sweeteners, such as maple syrup, brown rice syrup, honey, molasses, agave syrup, and stevia.

Q *What are trans fats and why are they so problematic for fibromyalgia patients?*

A During the process of making fats solid (hydrogenation) for use in margarine, trans fats and cis fats are created. These foreign fatty acids can be antagonistic to essential fatty acids (such as omega-3 and omega-6, found in fish oils) and contribute to inflammation by interfering with prostaglandin production. They are also known to lower your "good" high-density lipoprotein (HDL) cholesterol and raise your "bad" low-density lipoprotein (LDL) cholesterol.

Beverages

- Drink a minimum of 64 ounces (2 L) of spring, filtered, or reverse-osmosis water every day.
- Drink water at room temperature. Room-temperature water places less demand on your body because it does not require your body to heat or cool it to the same extent as cold or hot water.
- Enjoy herbal teas. Some can provide added health benefits. For example, chamomile tea helps calm the nervous system and can assist with sleep. Peppermint tea can assist with digestion. Green tea contains antioxidants.
- Add some lemon to your beverages for a mild detoxification and alkalinizing effect. A glass of lemon water is a great way to start the day.

Foundations of the Fibromyalgia Diet Program

- High protein
- Omega-3 rich
- Low carbohydrate
- Balanced
- Hypo-allergenic
- Organic
- Anti-inflammatory

Q *How much water should I drink every day?*

A You need to provide your body with ample water. Water makes up two-thirds of our core composition, and all of our organs depend on water to function properly. Water also allows us to flush out toxins. Chronic dehydration can cause the body to think it is hungry when in fact it is thirsty, and this can negatively impact our blood sugars. It can also contribute to constipation, decreasing elimination and further allowing toxins to accumulate. Staying well hydrated is therefore an important component of decreasing inflammation.. Our bodies can be too smart for our own good — when we are chronically dehydrated, our body tends to stop signaling to us that we are thirsty. You may need to retrain yourself. One big obstacle to drinking enough water with fibromyalgia is the frequency and urgency of urination that often plagues patients; however, avoiding water will only worsen this problem in the long term. From an Eastern medicine perspective, water is part of the yin that we need to nourish our bodies.

Q *Can I still drink wine or beer?*

A Alcohol acts as a depressant to the central nervous system and must be processed through the liver (which is likely already struggling with detoxification), and the fermentation process is not favorable if there is an underlying concern with yeast and sugars — for these reasons, alcohol can contribute to an increase in brain fog, low mood, pain, and other symptoms. Interestingly, from an Eastern medicine perspective, alcohol is also very damp-forming. Fibromyalgia is a condition that presents with damp stagnation.

CHAPTER 10
Menu Planning

> ## Case History
>
> *Slowly But Surely*
>
> Frank, a 43-year-old man, came to see us, complaining of symptoms, such as irritable bowl syndrome, widespread pain, and fatigue, plus sugar crashes following high-carbohydrate meals (with symptoms such as irritability, headaches, fatigue, and dizziness). After taking a detailed look at his diet, we suggested to Frank that he follow the fibromyalgia program strictly for 3 weeks. We made sure he was eating regularly and including protein with every meal, making choices that were both low-GI and low-GL foods. We suggested numerous shortcuts and encouraged him to phase in the diet gradually, starting with breakfast and working his way through each meal until all his meals followed the program.
>
> Frank noticed improvement in all of his symptoms after 2 weeks on the diet. By the end of week 3, Frank was still improving and began to notice small improvements in cognitive function, so he decided to stay on the diet longer than the initial 3 weeks planned. Frank continues to improve, slowly but steadily, and notices a decline in his health when he is unable to stick to his meal plans.

Menu plans and recipes can be easily built on the foundation of the fibromyalgia diet program. Here we provide you with four weeklong menu plans (28 days), including a shopping list for each week and a host of preparation tips for making food preparation even easier. The recipes listed in the menu plan can be found in the next chapter of this book, starting on page 159.

Implementing the Fibromyalgia Diet Program

❶ Determine nutritional status.
❷ Adopt USDA and Health Canada food guidelines.
❸ Isolate food groups to avoid.
❹ Choose organic foods.
❺ Eliminate allergenic and pro-inflammatory foods.
❻ Identify anti-inflammatory superfoods.
❼ Build menu plans that allow for easy preparation.
❽ Select recipes that meet daily nutrient requirements.

What Is a Menu Plan?

A menu plan enables you to use your recipes on a weekly or monthly basis, to generate shopping lists, and to ensure your meals are meeting your nutrient needs for good health.

How To Use a Menu Plan
Step 1
Read through the recipes for the week and highlight the ingredients you do not have in your pantry or refrigerator. Mark these missing ingredients on the shopping list. Plan ahead to get groceries. Remember to pace yourself. If you are the one who will be doing the shopping, make sure to schedule it in between rest periods. Take the shopping list with you to the grocery store or food market. If you find that shopping for a whole week is too much, try shopping for 1 week of breakfasts to get you started.

Step 2
Ask for assistance when possible (for example, ask a friend or family member to accompany you, ask someone to carry the groceries to your car, or arrange for their delivery). Many larger grocery stores provide scooters that you can borrow for free, and some will assign you a person to help put your food in the grocery cart. Many grocery chains will deliver food from their stores if you explain to the managers that you have a disability and find it difficult to shop. Some city services provide volunteers to do grocery shopping for a small fee, or sometimes for free if it is part of a charitable organization or church. In some larger cities, online grocery services will deliver to your door for a small fee (after you place your order with them using their website).

Step 3
Listen to your body and be mindful when eating. Before you were diagnosed with fibromyalgia, you probably rushed through your meals. Now you need to pace yourself as you eat, stopping and listening to what your body (not your mind) is telling you with regards to food. Stop and take a few deep belly breaths before beginning your meal to ensure your body is in the "rest and digest" parasympathetic state. Smell, observe, and chew your food well, tasting it with all your senses. Listen to how your body responds to the food.

Step 4

If you are doing an elimination diet to detect food intolerances, keep a diet diary and monitor symptoms when you reintroduce foods methodically.

Step 5

Follow the meal plans and enjoy the recipes!

Q *I'm overwhelmed at the thought of making all these changes at once. How can I cope?*

A If the thought of implementing these dietary changes and recommended meal plans all at once is too overwhelming and potentially draining, start by making changes to only one of the day's meals. For example, in week 1, put the focus only on breakfast. Ensure your breakfast follows the guidelines and use the meal plans only for breakfast. For the other meals and snacks, eat as you have been eating. Once you feel you have mastered breakfast, move on to lunch and so on.

Mentally Prepared

Week 1 Blues

During the first week, it is common to feel irritable and frustrated. This may be due to a combination of factors. Sugars and simple carbohydrates are easy go-to foods when you are fatigued. They provide the body with a quick source of energy and they are usually conveniently packaged. The problem is that they raise your blood sugar level quickly and then drop it. The last thing you need is a sugar crash and to have your cycles of reactive hypoglycemia further accentuated. Sugars also feed yeast, which has a loud, hungry voice in your body. As you starve out the yeast, you will feel irritated — but think of it as the yeast talking, not your body. It is also not uncommon to experience mild detoxification effects the first week. These effects can manifest with such symptoms as low-grade headaches and malaise.

Week 2 Prognosis

Despite this initial discomfort, the new diet starts to pay off. By the second week and onward, you should feel a noticeable reduction in symptoms. Our patients have often asked to stay on the fibromyalgia diet in the long term because they feel so much better. Stay the course and hang in until week 2 even if you do struggle at the start.

Weeks 3 and 4

After week 2, you won't need convincing. The results will be all the incentive you need to stick to this diet plan.

Handy Shopping Lists

We have broken down the grocery shopping week by week to keep it simpler for you. By week 2, you will have many of the grocery items in your pantry from week 1. Week 1 will be your biggest shopping trip. Ask for assistance with the grocery shopping if needed. Just give a friend, family member, or support person the list from this book.

Meal Preparation Shortcuts

Here are some tips to help decrease the amount of time you are on your feet preparing meals and to make cooking less overwhelming:

- Buy flash-frozen, precut vegetables.
- Buy organic baby food (fruits and vegetables) to use as sides and sauces to boost fruit and vegetable consumption.
- Make bigger batches of soups, casseroles, power bars, and other recipes to freeze for later use.
- Prepare extra proteins (for example, cook an extra chicken breast if you are having chicken for dinner), which can be used for lunch the next day.
- Make use of the slow cooker where indicated. Let it do the cooking for you while you sleep.
- Keep meal preparation and recipes simple by baking chicken breasts or fish, by steaming precut frozen veggies, and by using sauces made in large quantities to add flavor (refer to the sauces in the recipe section).
- Prepare all the ingredients for a smoothie the night before, and in the morning, all you have to do is blend and enjoy.
- Buy a sheet of clear acetate/transparency and a washable dry erase marker. Overlay the acetate on the recipe as you prepare a meal and check off the steps you have completed. This will enable you to keep track of the ingredients you have added to the recipe and avoid adding ingredients twice (for example, salt), helping you combat brain fog.
- Make a batch of pesto (see recipes, page 215) to use as a sauce for store-bought brown rice or quinoa pasta. Top with some chicken from the previous night's dinner!

Did You Know?

Meal Schedules

Make sure that you eat at regular intervals (never more than 4 hours between meals) to keep fuel coming into your body consistently, which will keep your energy higher and avoid the dips and valleys that result from skipping meals. Always eat first thing in the morning. This is ideal for your metabolism. If you wait to eat, you are sending your body the message that it is in starvation mode and it will slow your metabolism down to preserve energy. This can contribute to lethargy and weight gain.

About the Nutrient Analyses

Computer-assisted nutrient analysis of the meal plans and recipes was prepared by Kimberly Zammit, HBSc (the project supervisor was Len Piché, PhD, RD, Division of Food & Nutritional Sciences, Brescia University College, London, ON), using Food Processor® SQL, version 10.9, ESHA Research Inc., Salem OR (this software contains over 35,000 food items based largely on the latest USDA data and the entire Canadian Nutrient File, 2007b). The database was supplemented when necessary with data from the Canadian Nutrient File (version 2010) and documented data from other reliable sources.

The analysis was based on

- imperial weights and measures (except for foods typically packaged and used in metric quantities)
- the larger number of servings (i.e., the smaller portion) when there was a range
- the smaller ingredient quantity when there was a range
- the first ingredient listed when there was a choice of ingredients

Calculations involving meat and poultry use lean portions without skin and with visible fat trimmed. A pinch of salt was calculated as $\frac{1}{8}$ tsp (0.5 mL). All recipes were analyzed prior to cooking. Optional ingredients and garnishes, and ingredients that are not quantified, were not included in the calculations.

4-Week Meal Plans

Week 1 Grocery List

Many of these items may already be in your pantry and, if not, will continue to be used in subsequent weeks. Review the recipes listed in the Week 1 Meal Plan (page 144) to figure out how much you will need of each ingredient (amounts will depend on variables such as how many people you are cooking for at each meal, whether you are making extras for leftovers or future meals, whether you are halving or doubling a recipe, and so on.)

Whole Grains

❑ Brown rice
❑ Brown rice or quinoa pasta
❑ Gluten-free bread
❑ Millet
❑ Quinoa
❑ Quinoa flakes

Vegetables

❑ Baby spinach (see tip, below)
❑ Beets
❑ Broccoli
❑ Butternut squash (see tip, below)
❑ Carrots
❑ Celery
❑ Cucumber
❑ Garlic
❑ Gingerroot (see tip, below)
❑ Green beans
❑ Kale
❑ Onions (red and yellow)

Fruits

❑ Apples
❑ Fresh berries
❑ Frozen cherries or berries
❑ Haas avocado
❑ Kalamata olives
❑ Lemons

❑ Lemon juice (see tip, below)
❑ Lime juice

Fresh Herbs

❑ Basil
❑ Chives
❑ Dill
❑ Flat-leaf (Italian) parsley
❑ Oregano

Legumes

❑ Canned chickpeas
❑ Canned lentils
❑ Frozen lima beans

Meat and Fish

❑ Lean boneless lamb
❑ Boneless skinless chicken breasts
❑ Skinless farmed tilapia fillets (each about 6 oz/175 g)
❑ Skin-on trout fillets (each about 6 oz/175 g)

Nuts and Seeds

❑ Slivered raw almonds
❑ Whole raw almonds
❑ Raw cashews
❑ Raw walnut halves
❑ Almond butter
❑ Tahini

Oils and Vinegars

❑ Extra virgin olive oil
❑ Cider vinegar

Seasonings and Sweeteners

❑ *Spices:* black peppercorns, cayenne pepper, hot pepper flakes, ground cinnamon, ground cumin, poppy seeds
❑ *Dried herbs:* thyme
❑ Fine sea salt

☐ Almond extract

☐ Reduced-sodium ready-to-use vegetable broth

☐ Liquid honey

Beverages

☐ Plain almond milk

☐ Plain rice milk

☐ Coconut milk

☐ Apple juice

☐ Brown rice or hemp protein powder

Shopping and Storage Tips

- Buy prewashed organic baby spinach to minimize prep time.
- Buy precut butternut squash cubes to minimize prep time.
- Keep gingerroot in the freezer and grate from frozen as needed for longer shelf life.
- You can use bottled lemon or lime juice in any recipe that calls for it, but if you're feeling ambitious, freshly squeezed citrus juice has a superior flavor and no additives. If you want to use freshly squeezed juice, omit the bottled juice from this list and purchase limes and additional lemons.

Week 1 Make Aheads

- Make a batch of Hummus (page 169) on the previous Sunday night to use Monday through Wednesday; make another batch on Thursday night to use on Friday and Sunday.
- Make Lemon Vinaigrette (page 214) in advance for use throughout the week.
- Prepare smoothies in the blender container the night before, refrigerate, and blend in the morning. For the best consistency, wait to add any frozen ingredients until just before blending.
- Prepare the Creamy Morning Millet with Apples (page 164) on Friday night and let it cook overnight in the slow cooker, for an easy meal when you get up. Make enough to have leftovers for Sunday's breakfast too!
- The Walnut Quinoa Power Bars (page 168) will keep in the freezer for up to 6 months, so make a couple of batches on Saturday and freeze individual bars for easy snacks. Your future self will thank you!
- When making the Lemony Lentil Soup with Spinach (page 196) on Saturday and the Coconut-Spiked Pumpkin Soup with Cumin and Ginger (page 185) on Sunday, make a big enough batch that you have extras to freeze, for easy meals in the future. In general, soup can be stored in the freezer for up to 6 months.

Week 1 Meal Plan

Unless otherwise indicated, the amount given is 1 serving. The recipes (marked with an asterisk) can be found in Part 4. Each day emphasizes a particular nutrient boost for

	Monday	Tuesday	Wednesday	
Breakfast	Super Antioxidant Smoothie,* with 2 tbsp (30 mL) brown rice or hemp protein powder ½ avocado	2 slices toasted gluten-free bread, spread with 1 to 2 tbsp (15 to 30 mL) almond butter 1 apple	Super Antioxidant Smoothie,* with 2 tbsp (30 mL) brown rice or hemp protein powder and 2 tbsp (30 mL) ground chia or Salba	
Snack	½ cup (125 mL) Hummus* 8 brown rice crackers	½ cup (125 mL) berries 8 raw walnut halves	1 apple 12 raw almonds	
Lunch	Broiled Herbed Trout Fillets* 1 cup (250 mL) steamed spinach with 1 tbsp (15 mL) Lemon Vinaigrette*	Leftover chicken from Monday dinner Quick Sautéed Kale* 1 cup (250 mL) cooked brown rice	Leftover stir-fry from Tuesday dinner 1 avocado	
Snack	½ cup (125 mL) berries 12 raw almonds	¼ cup (60 mL) Hummus* 6 broccoli spears 2 carrot sticks	½ cup (125 mL) Hummus* 6 broccoli spears 2 carrot sticks	
Dinner	Apple Harvest Chicken* (make enough for leftovers) 1 cup (250 mL) brown rice pasta or quinoa pasta 1 cup (250 mL) steamed broccoli	Quinoa Vegetable Stir-Fry* (make enough for leftovers)	Grilled Garlic-Ginger Chicken Breasts* (make enough for leftovers) Roasted Beets with Carrots* 1 cup (250 mL) cooked brown rice	
Nutrient Boost	Omega-3 EFAs (from the trout)	Calcium (from the almonds, kale and broccoli)	Omega-3 EFAs and manganese (from the chia or Salba)	
Nutrient Analysis	Calories: 1356 Fat: 61 g Carbohydrate: 133 g Fiber: 31 g Protein: 74 g Calcium: 274 mg Iron: 10.6 mg	Calories: 1481 Fat: 41 g Carbohydrate: 231 g Fiber: 33 g Protein: 57 g Calcium: 505 mg Iron: 13.8 mg	Calories: 1347 Fat: 65 g Carbohydrate: 206 g Fiber: 52 g Protein: 45 g Calcium: 454 mg Iron: 12.2 mg	

treating fibromyalgia symptoms. The daily nutrient analysis shows how the menu meets the recommended daily allowances for key nutrients.

Thursday	Friday	Saturday	Sunday
Lemon water on rising 2 slices toasted gluten-free bread, spread with 1 to 2 tbsp (15 to 30 mL) almond butter 1 apple	Super Antioxidant Smoothie,* with 2 tbsp (30 mL) brown rice or hemp protein powder	Creamy Morning Millet with Apples* (make enough for leftovers) 12 raw almonds	Leftover Morning Millet from Saturday breakfast 12 raw almonds
½ cup (125 mL) berries 8 raw cashews	¼ cup (60 mL) Hummus* 6 broccoli spears 2 carrot sticks	1 Walnut Quinoa Power Bar*	½ cup (125 mL) berries 12 raw almonds
Leftover chicken from Wednesday dinner Spinach with Almonds*	Leftover tilapia from Thursday dinner 1 cup (250 mL) baby spinach with 1 tbsp (15 mL) Lemon Vinaigrette*	Lemony Lentil Soup with Spinach*	Coconut-Spiked Pumpkin Soup with Cumin and Ginger,* made with butternut squash
1 apple 12 raw almonds	1 apple 12 raw almonds	½ cup (125 mL) berries 8 raw cashews	¼ cup (60 mL) Hummus* 6 broccoli spears 2 carrot sticks
Lemon Dill Tilapia in Foil* (make enough for leftovers) Carrot and Ginger Salad* 1 cup (250 mL) cooked quinoa	1 cup (250 mL) brown rice or quinoa pasta with 2 tbsp (30 mL) Basil Pesto Sauce* 1 cup (250 mL) baby spinach with 1 tbsp (15 mL) Lemon Vinaigrette* ½ cup (125 mL) blueberries	Broiled Herbed Trout Fillets* Green Beans with Cashews*	Lamb Souvlaki* (make enough for leftovers) ½ cup (125 mL) sliced cucumber topped with 1 tbsp (15 mL) Lemon Vinaigrette* 1 cup (250 mL) cooked brown rice
Vitamin C (from the lemon water)	Vitamin B$_{12}$ (from the fish and nuts)	Magnesium (from the fish and almonds)	Iron (from the lamb)
Calories: 1513 Fat: 56 g Carbohydrate: 174 g Fiber: 29 g Protein: 90 g Calcium: 379 mg Iron: 11.3 mg	Calories: 1477 Fat: 80 g Carbohydrate: 136 g Fiber: 33 g Protein: 69 g Calcium: 609 mg Iron: 11.4 mg	Calories: 1635 Fat: 56 g Carbohydrate: 210 g Fiber: 36 g Protein: 83 g Calcium: 600 mg Iron: 16.2 mg	Calories: 1511 Fat: 71 g Carbohydrate: 173 g Fiber: 24 g Protein: 59 g Calcium: 454 mg Iron: 11.1 mg

Week 2 Grocery List

Cross off what you still have left from last week or already have in your pantry or fridge. Replenish any items you're running low on. Review the recipes listed in the Week 2 Meal Plan (page 148) to figure out how much you will need of each ingredient (amounts will depend on variables such as how many people you are cooking for at each meal, whether you are making extras for leftovers or future meals, whether you are halving or doubling a recipe, and so on.)

Whole Grains

- ❏ Brown rice
- ❏ Brown rice cakes
- ❏ Gluten-free dry bread crumbs
- ❏ Gluten-free bread
- ❏ Gluten-free large-flake (old-fashioned) rolled oats
- ❏ Quinoa
- ❏ Rice crackers

Vegetables

- ❏ Baby spinach (see tip, page 143)
- ❏ Carrots
- ❏ Celery
- ❏ Cucumber
- ❏ Garlic
- ❏ Gingerroot (see tip, page 143)
- ❏ Green beans
- ❏ Onions (red and yellow)
- ❏ Sweet potatoes
- ❏ Swiss chard
- ❏ Zucchini

Fruits

- ❏ Apples
- ❏ Dried apricots
- ❏ Fresh berries
- ❏ Frozen cherries or berries
- ❏ Hass avocados
- ❏ Kalamata olives
- ❏ Lemons
- ❏ Lemon juice (see tip, page 143)
- ❏ Lime juice
- ❏ Pomegranate

Fresh Herbs

- ❏ Cilantro
- ❏ Flat-leaf (Italian) parsley
- ❏ Mint
- ❏ Thyme

Legumes

- ❏ Canned cannellini (white kidney) beans
- ❏ Canned chickpeas
- ❏ Dried brown or green lentils

Meat and Fish

- ❏ 2 whole roasting chickens (each 5 to 6 lbs/2.5 to 3 kg)
- ❏ Skinless halibut steaks
- ❏ Skinless salmon fillets (each about 4 oz/125 g)

Nuts and Seeds

- ❏ Raw cashews
- ❏ Sesame seeds
- ❏ Raw sunflower seeds
- ❏ Ground flax seeds (flaxseed meal)
- ❏ Almond butter
- ❏ Tahini

Oils and Vinegars

- ❏ Extra virgin olive oil
- ❏ Cider vinegar

Seasonings and Sweeteners

- ❏ *Spices:* black peppercorns, cayenne pepper, cinnamon sticks, cumin seeds, dried Italian seasoning, ground cinnamon, ground coriander, ground cumin, ground turmeric, mild curry powder, poppy seeds

❑ Fine sea salt
❑ Reduced-sodium ready-to-use vegetable broth
❑ Dairy-free basil pesto
❑ Pure maple syrup
❑ Liquid honey

Beverages

❑ Plain almond milk
❑ Light coconut milk
❑ Brown rice or hemp protein powder

Week 2 Make Aheads

- Prepare Overnight Oatmeal (page 162) on Sunday, Tuesday and Thursday nights to enjoy Monday, Wednesday and Friday mornings.
- Make a batch of Hummus (page 169) on the previous Sunday night to use Monday and Wednesday.
- You can substitute store-bought guacamole in place of homemade Bolivian Guacamole (page 172) to reduce time on your feet preparing food. Make sure to read the ingredients.
- Remember to pull a Walnut Quinoa Power Bar (page 168) out of the freezer and let it thaw for at least an hour before your Tuesday morning snack.
- Be sure to make enough Sweet Potato and Spinach Curry with Quinoa (page 233) on Wednesday night that you have enough for both Thursday lunch and to freeze and reheat for Sunday dinner.
- When cooking quinoa for Thursday dinner, make an extra 3 cups (750 mL) cooked quinoa (that's 1 cup/250 mL raw) to use in the Pomegranate and Quinoa Salad with Sunflower Seeds (page 211) for Friday lunch. Refrigerate it in an airtight container overnight. Skip step 1 of the salad recipe and use the chilled quinoa in step 3.
- When making the Swiss Chard, Sweet Potato and Quinoa Soup (page 192) on Saturday, make a big enough batch that you have extras to freeze, for easy meals in the future. In general, soup can be stored in the freezer for up to 6 months.
- The Garlicky White Bean Spread (page 171) you make for your afternoon snack on Sunday will also be used on Monday and Wednesday in week 3, so make sure to prepare enough.

Week 2 Meal Plan

Unless otherwise indicated, the amount given is 1 serving. The recipes (marked with an asterisk) can be found in Part 4. Each day emphasizes a particular nutrient boost for

	Monday	Tuesday	Wednesday	
Breakfast	Overnight Oatmeal* ½ cup (125 mL) berries 1 to 2 tbsp (15 to 30 mL) sesame seeds	2 slices toasted gluten-free bread, spread with 1 to 2 tbsp (15 to 30 mL) almond butter 1 apple	Overnight Oatmeal* ½ cup (125 mL) berries 1 to 2 tbsp (15 to 30 mL) sesame seeds	
Snack	½ cup (125 mL) Hummus* 12 celery sticks	1 Walnut Quinoa Power Bar* (frozen from week 1)	¼ cup (60 mL) Hummus* 12 celery sticks	
Lunch	Leftover souvlaki from Sunday dinner 1 cup (250 mL) sliced cucumber, sprinkled with fresh mint	Leftover lentils from Monday dinner	Leftover chicken breast from Tuesday dinner Carrot and Ginger Salad*	
Snack	¼ cup (60 mL) Bolivian Guacamole* 12 rice crackers	½ cup (125 mL) berries	¼ cup (60 mL) Bolivian Guacamole* 8 rice crackers	
Dinner	Indian-Spiced Lentils with Peppery Apricots* (make enough for leftovers) 1 cup (250 mL) cooked brown rice	Lemon-Thyme Roast Chicken* (save some breast meat for Wednesday lunch) Sautéed Swiss Chard*	Sweet Potato and Spinach Curry with Quinoa* (make enough for leftovers and to freeze)	
Nutrient Boost	Vitamin B₅ (from the avocado)	Potassium (from the Swiss chard)	Arginine (from the almond butter and chicken)	
Nutrient Analysis	Calories: 1798 Fat: 69 g Carbohydrate: 235 g Fiber: 49 g Protein: 79 g Calcium: 667 mg Iron: 16.3 mg	Calories: 1368 Fat: 45 g Carbohydrate: 197 g Fiber: 30 g Protein: 59 g Calcium: 354 mg Iron: 14.5 mg	Calories: 1483 Fat: 73 g Carbohydrate: 167 g Fiber: 38 g Protein: 58 g Calcium: 558 mg Iron: 13.8 mg	

treating fibromyalgia symptoms. The daily nutrient analysis shows how the menu meets the recommended daily allowances for key nutrients.

Thursday	Friday	Saturday	Sunday
Super Antioxidant Smoothie,* with 2 tbsp (30 mL) brown rice or hemp protein powder	Overnight Oatmeal* ½ cup (125 mL) berries 1 to 2 tbsp (15 to 30 mL) sesame seeds	Toasted Quinoa Porridge*	Toasted Quinoa Porridge*
1 brown rice cake with 1 tbsp (15 mL) almond butter	1 apple	1 Walnut Quinoa Power Bar* (frozen from week 1) ½ cup (125 mL) berries	1 apple 8 raw almonds
Leftover curry from Wednesday dinner	Pomegranate and Quinoa Salad with Sunflower Seeds*	Swiss Chard, Sweet Potato and Quinoa Soup*	Leftover chicken breast from Saturday dinner Roasted Root Veggies*
1 apple 1 tbsp (15 mL) sesame seeds	Sandwich made with 2 brown rice cakes, ¼ avocado and 1 tbsp (15 mL) almond butter	1 apple with 1 tbsp (15 mL) almond butter	½ cup (125 mL) Garlicky White Bean Spread* 2 brown rice cakes
Cumin-Crusted Halibut Steaks* Green Beans with Cashews* ¼ to ½ cup (60 to 125 mL) cooked quinoa	Maple Ginger Salmon* Sautéed Swiss Chard* 1 cup (250 mL) cooked brown rice	Lemon-Thyme Roast Chicken* (save some breast meat for Sunday lunch) Stuffed Zucchini*	Sweet Potato and Spinach Curry with Quinoa* (frozen from Wednesday dinner; thaw and reheat)
Vitamin D_3 (from the halibut)	Selenium (from the Swiss chard)	Carnitine (from the chicken)	Vitamin B_1 (from the legumes)
Calories: 1562 Fat: 52 g Carbohydrate: 210 g Fiber: 46 g Protein: 77 g Calcium: 439 mg Iron: 21.4 mg	Calories: 1490 Fat: 54 g Carbohydrate: 209 g Fiber: 30 g Protein: 56 g Calcium: 488 mg Iron: 11.7 mg	Calories: 1365 Fat: 63 g Carbohydrate: 167 g Fiber: 24 g Protein: 60 g Calcium: 352 mg Iron: 16.8 mg	Calories: 1395 Fat: 54 g Carbohydrate: 185 g Fiber: 28 g Protein: 55 g Calcium: 301 mg Iron: 13.4 mg

Week 3 Grocery List

Cross off what you still have left from last week or already have in your pantry or fridge. Replenish any items you're running low on. Review the recipes listed in the Week 3 Meal Plan (page 152) to figure out how much you will need of each ingredient (amounts will depend on variables such as how many people you are cooking for at each meal, whether you are making extras for leftovers or future meals, whether you are halving or doubling a recipe, and so on.)

Whole Grains

- ❑ Amaranth
- ❑ Brown rice
- ❑ Brown rice or quinoa pasta
- ❑ Brown rice cakes
- ❑ 8-inch (20 cm) rice paper rounds
- ❑ Gluten-free bread
- ❑ Millet
- ❑ Quinoa
- ❑ Quinoa flakes

Vegetables

- ❑ Baby spinach (see tip, page 143)
- ❑ Beets
- ❑ Broccoli
- ❑ Butternut squash (see tip, page 143)
- ❑ Carrots
- ❑ Garlic
- ❑ Gingerroot (see tip, page 143)
- ❑ Green onions
- ❑ Onions
- ❑ Parsnips
- ❑ Sweet potatoes
- ❑ Swiss chard
- ❑ Turnips

Fruits

- ❑ Apples
- ❑ Fresh berries
- ❑ Frozen cherries or berries
- ❑ Haas avocado
- ❑ Lemons
- ❑ Lemon juice (see tip, page 143)
- ❑ Limes
- ❑ Lime juice (see tip, page 143)
- ❑ Pomegranate seeds

Fresh Herbs

- ❑ Basil
- ❑ Cilantro
- ❑ Dill
- ❑ Mint
- ❑ Oregano
- ❑ Sage
- ❑ Thyme

Legumes

- ❑ Canned chickpeas
- ❑ Dried brown or green lentils

Meat and Fish

- ❑ Butterflied leg of lamb (2 lbs/1 kg)
- ❑ Extra-lean ground lamb
- ❑ Boneless skinless chicken breasts
- ❑ Skinless Pacific halibut fillets (each about 5 oz/150 g)
- ❑ Skinless salmon fillet (about 1½ lbs/750 g total)

Nuts and Seeds

- ❑ Raw almonds
- ❑ Raw cashews
- ❑ Raw walnut halves
- ❑ Pine nuts
- ❑ Sesame seeds
- ❑ Almond butter

Oils and Vinegars

- ❑ Extra virgin olive oil
- ❑ Coconut oil
- ❑ Cider vinegar

Seasonings and Sweeteners

❏ *Spices:* black peppercorns, cayenne pepper, cinnamon sticks, coriander seeds, cumin seeds, garam masala, ground cardamom, ground cinnamon, ground coriander, ground cumin, ground nutmeg, ground turmeric

❏ *Dried herbs:* oregano, parsley

❏ Fine sea salt

❏ Tamari

❏ Reduced-sodium ready-to-use vegetable broth

❏ Liquid honey

Beverages

❏ Plain almond milk

❏ Light coconut milk

❏ Brown rice or hemp protein powder

Energy-Saving Prep Tips

- Purchase precut vegetables whenever possible, or precut your own when you have the time and energy, then freeze them for future use.
- Cook a large batch of legumes and freeze them in individual portions, so you have them on hand to add to soups, salads and other dishes. Thaw overnight in the refrigerator before use.
- Use Lemon Vinaigrette (page 214) as a topping or sauce for a simple baked chicken breast or steamed veggies — delicious!

- Use a slow cooker to prepare your meals whenever possible, to reduce time on your feet cooking.
- Whenever you can, make extras and freeze them for easy future meals.

Week 3 Make Aheads

- The Garlicky White Bean Spread (page 171) for your afternoon snack on Monday and Wednesday is already made, thanks to your Sunday afternoon snack in Week 2.
- On Tuesday morning, make enough of the Indian Carrot and Quinoa Porridge (page 166) to have leftovers for Wednesday and Thursday breakfast too.
- On Wednesday night, bake extra chicken breasts for Thursday and Friday lunches.
- Prepare Hot Millet Amaranth Cereal (page 165) on Friday and Saturday nights and let it cook overnight in the slow cooker, for easy meals when you get up on Saturday and Sunday.
- When making the Curry-Roasted Squash and Apple Soup (page 190) on Sunday, make a big enough batch that you have extras to freeze, for easy meals in the future. In general, soup can be stored in the freezer for up to 6 months.
- Remember to pull a Walnut Quinoa Power Bar (page 168) out of the freezer and let it thaw for at least an hour before your Sunday afternoon snack.

Week 3 Meal Plan

Unless otherwise indicated, the amount given is 1 serving. The recipes (marked with an asterisk) can be found in Part 4. Each day emphasizes a particular nutrient boost for

	Monday	Tuesday	Wednesday	
Breakfast	Super Antioxidant Smoothie,* with 2 tbsp (30 mL) brown rice or hemp protein powder	Indian Carrot and Quinoa Porridge* (make enough for leftovers)	Leftover porridge from Tuesday breakfast	
Snack	1 apple with 1 tbsp (15 mL) almond butter	½ cup (125 mL) berries 8 raw walnut halves	1 apple with 1 tbsp (15 mL) almond butter	
Lunch	Salmon Wraps* ½ cup (125 mL) steamed broccoli florets, sprinkled with sea salt ½ avocado	Leftover lamb dish from Monday dinner ½ avocado	Swiss Chard, Sweet Potato and Quinoa Soup* (frozen from week 2; thaw and reheat)	
Snack	½ cup (125 mL) Garlicky White Bean Spread* (from Sunday week 2) 2 brown rice cakes	½ cup (125 mL) berries	½ cup (125 mL) Garlicky White Bean Spread* 2 brown rice cakes	
Dinner	Middle Eastern Lamb, Greens and Quinoa* (make enough for leftovers)	Halibut with Coconut Lime Sauce* 1 cup (250 mL) steamed kale or spinach ¾ cup (175 mL) brown rice or quinoa pasta	4-oz (125 g) boneless skinless chicken breast, drizzled with 1 tbsp (15 mL) Lemon Vinaigrette* and baked Sautéed Spinach with Pine Nuts*	
Nutrient Boost	Iodine (from the sea salt)	Tryptophan (from the halibut)	Vitamin B_2 (from the spinach and nuts)	
Nutrient Analysis	Calories: 1400 Fat: 59 g Carbohydrate: 157 g Fiber: 37 g Protein: 75 g Calcium: 395 mg Iron: 13.7 mg	Calories: 1426 Fat: 56 g Carbohydrate: 174 g Fiber: 31 g Protein: 68 g Calcium: 380 mg Iron: 11.1 mg	Calories: 1504 Fat: 59 g Carbohydrate: 181 g Fiber: 28 g Protein: 74 g Calcium: 427 mg Iron: 12.9 mg	

treating fibromyalgia symptoms. The daily nutrient analysis shows how the menu meets the recommended daily allowances for key nutrients.

Thursday	Friday	Saturday	Sunday
Leftover porridge from Tuesday breakfast	2 slices toasted gluten-free bread, spread with 1 to 2 tbsp (15 to 30 mL) almond butter 1 apple	Hot Millet Amaranth Cereal* ½ cup (125 mL) berries	Hot Millet Amaranth Cereal* ½ cup (125 mL) berries
½ cup (125 mL) berries 8 raw walnut halves	½ cup (125 mL) berries 8 raw walnut halves	1 apple 12 raw almonds	1 apple 12 raw almonds
Autumn Harvest Salad and Harvest Dressing* Leftover chicken breast from Wednesday dinner	Herbed Chicken and Pomegranate Salad,* made with leftover chicken breast from Wednesday dinner	Leftover curry from Friday dinner 1 slice gluten-free toast	Curry-Roasted Squash and Apple Soup* 2 slices gluten-free toast
½ cup (125 mL) berries 8 raw walnut halves	1 brown rice cake with 1 tbsp (15 mL) almond butter	1 apple with 1 tbsp (15 mL) almond butter	Walnut Quinoa Power Bar* (frozen from week 1)
Swiss Chard, Sweet Potato and Quinoa Soup* (frozen from week 2; thaw and reheat)	Vegetable Curry with Lentils and Spinach* (make enough for leftovers)	BBQ Butterflied Leg of Lamb* 1 cup (250 mL) baby spinach with 1 tbsp (15 mL) Lemon Vinaigrette* 1 cup (250 mL) cooked brown rice	Grilled Chicken Kabobs* (make enough for leftovers) 1 cup (250 mL) cooked quinoa 1 cup (250 mL) chopped carrots and broccoli (raw or steamed)
Vitamin B$_6$ (from the chicken)	Antioxidant vitamin C (from the berries)	Iron (from the amaranth, lamb and lentils)	Copper (from the quinoa and walnuts)
Calories: 1408 Fat: 78 g Carbohydrate: 122 g Fiber: 20 g Protein: 67 g Calcium: 336 mg Iron: 9.7 mg	Calories: 1408 Fat: 52 g Carbohydrate: 200 g Fiber: 33 g Protein: 49 g Calcium: 300 mg Iron: 11.9 mg	Calories: 1465 Fat: 64 g Carbohydrate: 188 g Fiber: 25 g Protein: 62 g Calcium: 352 mg Iron: 17.5 mg	Calories: 1502 Fat: 46 g Carbohydrate: 224 g Fiber: 31 g Protein: 60 g Calcium: 320 mg Iron: 12.3 mg

Week 4 Grocery List

You likely have a lot of this in your pantry or fridge by now from previous weeks. Replenish any items you're running low on. Review the recipes listed in the Week 4 Meal Plan (page 156) to figure out how much you will need of each ingredient (amounts will depend on variables such as how many people you are cooking for at each meal, whether you are making extras for leftovers or future meals, whether you are halving or doubling a recipe, and so on.)

Whole Grains

- ❑ Brown rice
- ❑ Brown rice cakes
- ❑ Gluten-free bread
- ❑ Gluten-free cracker crumbs
- ❑ Gluten-free steel-cut oats
- ❑ Quinoa

Vegetables

- ❑ Baby spinach (see tip, page 143)
- ❑ Beets
- ❑ Broccoli
- ❑ Carrots
- ❑ Celery
- ❑ Garlic
- ❑ Gingerroot (see tip, page 143)
- ❑ Green beans
- ❑ Green onions
- ❑ Leeks
- ❑ Parsnips
- ❑ Onions (red and yellow)
- ❑ Frozen spinach cubes
- ❑ Turnips
- ❑ Zucchini

Fruits

- ❑ Apples
- ❑ Fresh berries
- ❑ Frozen cherries or berries
- ❑ Hass avocados
- ❑ Lemons
- ❑ Lemon juice (see tip, page 143)
- ❑ Peaches
- ❑ Ruby red grapefruits

Fresh Herbs

- ❑ Basil
- ❑ Chives
- ❑ Cilantro
- ❑ Mint
- ❑ Oregano
- ❑ Parsley
- ❑ Sage
- ❑ Thyme

Legumes

- ❑ Canned chickpeas
- ❑ Canned lentils
- ❑ Dried red lentils

Meat and Fish

- ❑ Roasting chicken (about 3 lbs/1.5 kg)
- ❑ Chicken pieces (drumsticks or breasts)
- ❑ Skinless salmon fillets
- ❑ Skinless sole fillets (each about 3 1/2 oz/100 g)
- ❑ Canned wild salmon (6-oz/170 g cans)

Nuts and Seeds

- ❑ Slivered raw almonds
- ❑ Raw cashews
- ❑ Raw pecan halves
- ❑ Raw walnut halves
- ❑ Sesame seeds
- ❑ Almond butter

Oils and Vinegars

- ❑ Coconut oil
- ❑ Cider vinegar
- ❑ Rice vinegar
- ❑ Extra virgin olive oil

Seasonings and Sweeteners

- *Spices:* black peppercorns, cinnamon sticks, garam masala, ground cardamom, ground coriander, ground cumin, ground nutmeg, ground turmeric, poppy seeds
- *Dried herbs:* bay leaves
- Fine sea salt
- Tamari
- Dijon mustard
- Reduced-sodium ready-to-use vegetable broth
- Reduced-sodium ready-to-use chicken broth
- Liquid honey
- Pure maple syrup

Beverages

- Plain almond milk
- Coconut milk
- Brown rice or hemp protein powder

Week 4 Make Aheads

- Remember to pull a Walnut Quinoa Power Bar (page 168) out of the freezer and let it thaw for at least an hour before your Monday morning and Tuesday and Wednesday afternoon snacks.
- Prepare the Irish Oatmeal (page 163) on Monday night and let it cook overnight in the slow cooker, for an easy meal when you get up on Tuesday.
- On Friday morning, make enough of the Indian Carrot and Quinoa Porridge (page 166) to have leftovers for Saturday and Sunday breakfast too.
- When making the Lentil and Spinach Soup (page 195) on Wednesday and the Winter Soup Purée (page 193) on Sunday, make big enough batches that you have extras to freeze, for easy meals in the future. In general, soup can be stored in the freezer for up to 6 months.

Note

Over the course of 4 weeks, we have introduced a substantial number of new recipes. If you find this meal plan overwhelming, add only one or two new recipes per week. Once you are familiar with a recipe, it will be easier to prepare and you will figure out shortcuts that work for you. Once you are ready for more variety, or if any of the meals chosen here don't appeal to you, structure your meals along these guidelines and enjoy the other recipes included in Part 4.

Week 4 Meal Plan

Unless otherwise indicated, the amount given is 1 serving. The recipes (marked with an asterisk) can be found in Part 4. Each day emphasizes a particular nutrient boost for

	Monday	Tuesday	Wednesday	
Breakfast	Super Antioxidant Smoothie,* with 2 tbsp (30 mL) brown rice or hemp protein powder	Irish Oatmeal*	Super Antioxidant Smoothie,* with 2 tbsp (30 mL) brown rice or hemp protein powder and 1 tbsp (15 mL) spirulina	
Snack	Walnut Quinoa Power Bar* (frozen from week 1) 1 apple	12 celery sticks with 1 tbsp (15 mL) almond butter	1 peach 8 pecan halves	
Lunch	Moroccan Lentil Soup* 2 slices gluten-free toast	Curry-Roasted Squash and Apple Soup* (frozen from week 3; thaw and reheat)	Lentil and Spinach Soup* 6-oz (170 g) can wild salmon 2 slices gluten-free toast	
Snack	1 brown rice cake with 1 tbsp (15 mL) almond butter	Walnut Quinoa Power Bar* (frozen from week 1) ½ cup (125 mL) berries	Walnut Quinoa Power Bar* (frozen from week 1) 1 apple	
Dinner	Leftover chicken kabobs from Sunday dinner Spinach with Almonds*	Fish for the Sole* Green Beans with Cashews*	Baked Chicken with Lemon Herb Sauce* (make enough for leftovers) Stuffed Zucchini*	
Nutrient Boost	Antioxidant vitamin C (from the smoothie)	Potassium (from the squash)	Tyrosine (from the spirulina)	
Nutrient Analysis	Calories: 1578 Fat: 53 g Carbohydrate: 213 g Fiber: 38 g Protein: 75 g Calcium: 358 mg Iron: 15.9 mg	Calories: 1482 Fat: 53 g Carbohydrate: 193 g Fiber: 39 g Protein: 73 g Calcium: 534 mg Iron: 15.8 mg	Calories: 1575 Fat: 58 g Carbohydrate: 187 g Fiber: 35 g Protein: 94 g Calcium: 520 mg Iron: 17.7 mg	

treating fibromyalgia symptoms. The daily nutrient analysis shows how the menu meets the recommended daily allowances for key nutrients.

Thursday	Friday	Saturday	Sunday
2 slices toasted gluten-free bread, spread with 1 to 2 tbsp (15 to 30 mL) almond butter 1 apple	Indian Carrot and Quinoa Porridge* (make enough for leftovers)	Leftover porridge from Friday breakfast	Leftover porridge from Friday breakfast
1 peach 8 walnut halves	1 apple 8 pecan halves	½ cup (125 mL) berries 10 to 12 raw almonds	1 apple 8 walnut halves
Avocado, Grapefruit and Quinoa Salad* 2 medium carrots	Red Lentil Curry with Coconut and Cilantro (make enough for leftovers) 1 cup (250 mL) cooked brown rice	Autumn Harvest Salad and Harvest Dressing,* topped with 1 cup (250 mL) chickpeas or a 6-oz (170 g) can wild salmon	Winter Soup Purée* Leftover chicken breast from Saturday dinner
1 brown rice cake with 1 tbsp (15 mL) almond butter	½ cup (125 mL) berries 8 walnut halves	1 brown rice cake with 1 tbsp (15 mL) almond butter	12 celery sticks with 1 tbsp (15 mL) almond butter
Leftover chicken from Wednesday dinner 1 cup (250 mL) steamed spinach 1 cup (250 mL) cooked brown rice	Maple Ginger Salmon* 1 cup (250 mL) steamed vegetables ½ cup (125 mL) cooked quinoa	Roast Chicken with Leeks* (save some breast meat for Sunday lunch) Green Beans with Cashews*	Leftover curry from Friday lunch Fragrant Coconut Rice*
Glutamine (from the chicken)	Methionine (from the salmon)	Lysine (from the salmon)	Manganese (from the lentils)
Calories: 1451 Fat: 55 g Carbohydrate: 207 g Fiber: 30 g Protein: 49 g Calcium: 296 mg Iron: 9.1 mg	Calories: 1492 Fat: 62 g Carbohydrate: 192 g Fiber: 27 g Protein: 51 g Calcium: 212 mg Iron: 9.7 mg	Calories: 1739 Fat: 68 g Carbohydrate: 210 g Fiber: 43 g Protein: 86 g Calcium: 428 mg Iron: 15.7 mg	Calories: 1531 Fat: 77 g Carbohydrate: 166 g Fiber: 30 g Protein: 62 g Calcium: 370 mg Iron: 13.0 mg

Part 4

100 Recipes

Introduction to the Recipes

Eating well is a challenge for many people, but particularly when you are struggling with fibromyalgia and dealing with such symptoms as chronic pain, brain fog and fatigue. With that in mind, we've provided you with a range of recipes that are easy to make and delicious. We hand-selected every recipe to give you options that are hypoallergenic and nutrient-rich.

Remember to pace yourself — try one new recipe each week. When you are ready, try following the entire meal plan as outlined in the previous chapter. Once you are comfortable with the meal plan, you can have some fun with it! Mix it up; try new things. All of these recipes have been developed with multiple food intolerances in mind.

Using these recipes to help you eat well can improve your symptoms and increase your overall well-being. Remember, change takes time. You have taken the first steps down the road to recovery, but you are bound to hit a few potholes.

We hope you enjoy these recipes as much as we do, and that mealtimes become a pleasurable experience for you again. Here's a toast to your health!

Breakfast, Snacks and Beverages

Overnight Oatmeal

Makes 2 servings

This easy-to-prepare breakfast is full of nutrients, including manganese, zinc and B vitamins such as thiamine (B_1), pantothenic acid (B_5), biotin, choline and PABA (para-aminobenzoic acid). Oatmeal is also filling, high in fiber and beneficial for lowering cholesterol.

Tip

Make sure to choose rolled oats that are certified gluten-free.

1 cup	large-flake (old-fashioned) rolled oats	250 mL
2 tbsp	ground flax seeds (flaxseed meal)	30 mL
1 cup	plain almond, rice or hemp milk	250 mL
½ tsp	vanilla extract	2 mL

Suggested Accompaniments

Warm or cold plain almond, rice or hemp milk

Fresh fruit, chopped nuts or seeds

1. In a medium bowl, combine oats, flax seeds, milk and vanilla. Cover and refrigerate overnight.

2. Serve cold or microwave on Medium (50%) for 1 to 2 minutes or until warm. Top with any of the suggested accompaniments, as desired.

Nutrients per serving	
Calories	232
Fat	6 g
Carbohydrate	35 g
Fiber	6 g
Protein	11 g
Calcium	176 mg
Iron	2.2 mg

Irish Oatmeal

Steel-cut oats have more flavor than rolled oats and an appealingly crunchy texture.

Tips

Make sure to choose steel-cut oats that are certified gluten-free.

Although it's a bit of work to prepare long-cooking whole-grain cereals, such as steel-cut oats, they can actually be quite convenient. Make a big batch on Sunday, cover and refrigerate leftovers. You can enjoy them throughout much of the week. When you're ready to serve, add a little water and cover. Reheat on the stovetop or in a microwave oven.

Nutrients per serving	
Calories	60
Fat	1 g
Carbohydrate	11 g
Fiber	1 g
Protein	2 g
Calcium	3 mg
Iron	0.6 mg

4 cups	water	1 L
½ tsp	salt	2 mL
1 cup	steel-cut oats	250 mL

Suggested Accompaniments

Maple syrup or honey

Chopped nuts or seeds

Plain almond, rice or hemp milk

1. In a large saucepan over medium heat, bring water and salt to a boil. Gradually stir in oats and return to a boil. Reduce heat to low, cover and simmer, stirring occasionally, until oats are tender, about 40 minutes. Serve with maple syrup, nuts and milk or non-dairy alternative, if using.

Variation

Slow Cooker Method: Use a small ($3\frac{1}{2}$ quart) lightly greased slow cooker. Combine ingredients in stoneware. Cover and cook on Low for 8 hours or overnight, or on High for 4 hours.

Creamy Morning Millet with Apples

Expand your nutritional range by enjoying millet as a cereal. Refrigerate leftovers for up to 2 days and reheat portions in the microwave.

Tips

If you prefer a non-creamy version, substitute water for the rice milk.

Use plain or vanilla-flavored rice milk. Vary the quantity to suit your preference. Three cups (750 mL) produces a firmer result. If you like your cereal to be creamy, use the larger quantity.

Nutrients per serving	
Calories	228
Fat	2 g
Carbohydrate	48 g
Fiber	6 g
Protein	4 g
Calcium	157 mg
Iron	1.1 mg

• **Small (3½ quart) slow cooker, stoneware greased**

1 cup	millet	250 mL
3 to 4 cups	enriched rice milk or water (see tips, at left)	750 mL to 1 L
3	apples, peeled, cored and chopped	3
¼ tsp	salt	1 mL

Suggested Accompaniments

Fresh berries

Chopped nuts

1. In prepared slow cooker stoneware, combine millet, rice milk, apples and salt. Cover and cook on High for 4 hours or on Low for 8 hours or overnight. Stir well, spoon into bowls and sprinkle with fruit and/or nuts, if using.

Variation

Use half millet and half short-grain brown rice.

Hot Millet Amaranth Cereal

Makes 6 servings

Here's a great way to start your day and add variety to your diet. Both millet and amaranth are relatively quick and easy to cook — so long as you keep the temperature low, they don't need to be stirred. Use a sweetener of your choice and add dried fruit and nuts as you please.

Tip

For best results, toast the millet and amaranth before cooking. Stir the grains in a dry skillet over medium heat until they crackle and release their aroma, about 5 minutes.

2½ cups	water	625 mL
½ cup	millet, toasted (see tip, at left)	125 mL
½ cup	amaranth	125 mL

Suggested Accompaniments

Plain almond, rice or hemp milk

Honey or maple syrup

Chopped nuts

1. In a saucepan over medium heat, bring water to a boil. Add millet and amaranth in a steady stream, stirring constantly. Return to a boil. Reduce heat to low. Cover and simmer until grains are tender and liquid is absorbed, about 25 minutes. Serve hot, sweetened to taste and with milk or non-dairy alternative. Sprinkle with nuts, if using.

Variation

Slow Cooker Method: Use a small (3½ quart) lightly greased slow cooker. Combine ingredients in stoneware, adding ½ cup (125 mL) additional water to mixture. Place a clean tea towel, folded in half (so you will have two layers), over top of the stoneware to absorb moisture. Cover and cook on Low for 8 hours or overnight, or on High for 4 hours.

Nutrients per serving	
Calories	124
Fat	2 g
Carbohydrate	23 g
Fiber	4 g
Protein	4 g
Calcium	29 mg
Iron	1.7 mg

Indian Carrot and Quinoa Porridge

Makes 4 servings

This delectable porridge is based on a popular Indian dessert, gajar halva.

Tip

Experiment with adding raw nuts instead of salted roasted nuts.

Make Ahead

Store the cooled porridge in an airtight container in the refrigerator for up to 3 days. Reheat individual portions in the microwave on High for 45 to 60 seconds or until warm, then sprinkle with pistachios.

12 oz	carrots, finely shredded (about 2½ cups/625 mL)	375 g
½ cup	quinoa, rinsed	125 mL
¾ tsp	ground cardamom	3 mL
¼ tsp	fine sea salt	1 mL
2½ cups	plain almond, rice, coconut or hemp milk	625 mL
1 cup	water	250 mL
¼ cup	liquid honey, brown rice syrup or agave nectar	60 mL
1 tbsp	coconut oil	15 mL
¼ cup	lightly salted roasted pistachios or cashews	60 mL

1. In a medium saucepan, combine carrots, quinoa, cardamom, salt, milk, water and honey. Bring to a gentle boil, stirring, over medium-high heat. Reduce heat and simmer, stirring occasionally, for 35 to 40 minutes or until carrots are very tender and mixture is thickened. Remove from heat and stir in coconut oil until blended. Let cool completely. Sprinkle with pistachios just before serving.

Nutrients per serving

Calories	294
Fat	10 g
Carbohydrate	47 g
Fiber	5 g
Protein	6 g
Calcium	55 mg
Iron	1.6 mg

Toasted Quinoa Porridge

Makes 2 servings

This power breakfast is an easy bowlful of deliciousness. Not as heavy as other grain porridges, it's one of those magical breakfast dishes that works for any season of the year.

½ cup	quinoa, rinsed	125 mL
½ tsp	ground cinnamon	2 mL
⅛ tsp	fine sea salt	0.5 mL
1¼ cups	plain almond, rice, coconut or hemp milk, divided	300 mL
1 cup	water	250 mL

Suggested Accompaniments

Agave nectar, honey, brown rice syrup or pure maple syrup

Fresh fruit

1. In a small saucepan, over medium heat, toast quinoa, stirring, for 2 to 3 minutes or until golden and fragrant. Add cinnamon, salt, 1 cup (250 mL) of the milk and water; bring to a boil. Reduce heat to low, cover and simmer, stirring occasionally, for about 25 minutes or until liquid is absorbed.

2. Serve drizzled with the remaining milk and any of the suggested accompaniments, as desired.

Nutrients per serving	
Calories	194
Fat	4 g
Carbohydrate	33 g
Fiber	4 g
Protein	7 g
Calcium	34 mg
Iron	2.2 mg

Walnut Quinoa Power Bars

Makes 8 bars

Together with walnuts and almond butter, quinoa flakes give these bars a major punch of protein power.

Tip

You can also roll the mixture into 1-inch (2.5 cm) balls instead of making bars.

Make Ahead

Store bars in an airtight container at room temperature for up to 1 week or in the refrigerator for up to 3 weeks. Or wrap them in plastic wrap, then foil, completely enclosing them, and freeze for up to 6 months. Let thaw at room temperature for 1 hour before serving.

Nutrients per bar

Calories	341
Fat	13 g
Carbohydrate	48 g
Fiber	5 g
Protein	10 g
Calcium	67 mg
Iron	2.6 mg

- 8-inch (20 cm) metal baking pan, lined with foil, sprayed with nonstick cooking spray

½ cup	brown rice syrup or liquid honey	125 mL
⅓ cup	unsweetened natural almond butter	75 mL
½ tsp	ground cinnamon	2 mL
⅛ tsp	fine sea salt	0.5 mL
½ tsp	almond extract	2 mL
2 cups	quinoa flakes	500 mL
½ cup	coarsely chopped toasted walnuts	125 mL

1. In a large bowl, whisk together brown rice syrup, almond butter, cinnamon, salt and almond extract until well blended. Stir in quinoa flakes and walnuts until just combined.

2. Press mixture into prepared pan. Refrigerate for 30 minutes. Using foil liner, lift mixture from pan and transfer to a cutting board. Peel off foil and cut into 8 bars.

Variations

Replace the quinoa flakes with quick-cooking rolled oats.

Any other nuts, or sunflower seeds, can be substituted for the walnuts.

Hummus

You can buy hummus, the classic spread from the Middle East, in most supermarkets, but it's so easy to make at home. Serve it as a dip with pita wedges or use as a sandwich spread.

• Food processor

1	can (19 oz/540 mL) chickpeas, rinsed and drained	1
⅓ cup	kalamata olives, pitted (about 12)	75 mL
¼ cup	water	60 mL
3 tbsp	freshly squeezed lemon juice	45 mL
2 tbsp	tahini	30 mL
2 tbsp	olive oil	30 mL
2	cloves garlic, chopped	2
¼ tsp	ground cumin (optional)	1 mL
2 tbsp	finely chopped fresh parsley	30 mL

1. In food processor, purée chickpeas, olives, water, lemon juice, tahini, olive oil, garlic and cumin (if using) until smooth.

2. Transfer to a bowl; stir in parsley. Cover and refrigerate.

Nutrients per ¼ cup (60 mL)

Calories	120
Fat	7 g
Carbohydrate	12 g
Fiber	3 g
Protein	4 g
Calcium	22 mg
Iron	0.9 mg

Tahini Dip

Serve this traditional Middle Eastern sesame dip with vegetable crudités or fried falafel, or on a salad of crispy lettuce, cucumber, tomatoes and onion.

Make Ahead

Prepare through step 1, transfer to a bowl, cover and refrigerate for up to 1 week. To serve, sprinkle with parsley and paprika.

• Blender

⅔ cup	tahini paste	150 mL
1	clove garlic, smashed	1
½ tsp	salt	2 mL
½ tsp	sweet paprika	2 mL
¼ tsp	cayenne pepper	1 mL
¼ tsp	ground cumin	1 mL
⅓ cup	freshly squeezed lemon juice	75 mL
½ cup	water (approx.)	125 mL

Garnish

2 tbsp	minced fresh parsley	30 mL
¼ tsp	paprika	1 mL

1. In blender, on low speed, blend tahini paste, garlic, salt, paprika, cayenne and cumin. With motor running, through hole in top, gradually pour in lemon juice and just enough water until desired consistency.

2. To serve, transfer to a bowl and sprinkle with parsley and paprika.

Nutrients per ¼ cup (60 mL)

Calories	234
Fat	20 g
Carbohydrate	11 g
Fiber	2 g
Protein	7 g
Calcium	62 mg
Iron	2.0 mg

Garlicky White Bean Spread

This spread makes a healthy and nutritious snack that is high in protein and full of nutrients, including vitamin B$_6$, vitamin C, magnesium, folate, choline and inositol.

Tips

If using a 19-oz (540 mL) can of beans, drain and measure out 1$\frac{2}{3}$ cups (400 mL) beans.

This spread may also be served as a dip.

Make Ahead

Store in an airtight container in the refrigerator for up to 3 days.

Nutrients per ¼ cup (60 mL)	
Calories	76
Fat	2 g
Carbohydrate	12 g
Fiber	3 g
Protein	4 g
Calcium	32 mg
Iron	1.0 mg

• **Food processor**

3	cloves garlic, minced	3
1	can (14 to 15 oz/398 to 425 mL) cannellini (white kidney) beans, drained and rinsed	1
⅔ cup	cooked quinoa, cooled	150 mL
1 tbsp	dried Italian seasoning	15 mL
½ tsp	fine sea salt	2 mL
¼ cup	freshly squeezed lemon juice	60 mL
1 tbsp	extra virgin olive oil	15 mL
¼ cup	packed fresh flat-leaf (Italian) parsley, chopped	60 mL

1. In food processor, combine garlic, beans, quinoa, Italian seasoning, salt, lemon juice and oil; process until smooth. Transfer to a serving dish and stir in parsley.

Bolivian Guacamole

Avocados and earthy quinoa — two Bolivian superfoods — join forces in this spin on guacamole. The emerald dip looks especially gorgeous when made with black or red quinoa.

3	firm-ripe Hass avocados, diced	3
½ cup	cooked red, black or white quinoa, cooled	125 mL
½ cup	packed fresh cilantro leaves, chopped	125 mL
¼ tsp	ground cumin	1 mL
Pinch	chipotle chile powder or cayenne pepper	Pinch
2 tbsp	freshly squeezed lime juice	30 mL
	Fine sea salt	

1. In a medium bowl, using a fork, combine avocados, quinoa, cilantro, cumin, chipotle chile powder and lime juice. Gently mash until guacamole is well blended but still slightly chunky. Season to taste with salt.

Nutrients per ¼ cup (60 mL)

Calories	174
Fat	15 g
Carbohydrate	11 g
Fiber	7 g
Protein	2 g
Calcium	15 mg
Iron	0.9 mg

Super Antioxidant Smoothie

Makes 2 servings

This smoothie recipe is an easy way to incorporate greens into your diet and get a healthy serving of the antioxidant vitamins C and E, which can help reduce the oxidative stress seen in fibromyalgia.

Tips

Experiment with adding brown rice protein powder to the smoothie.

In addition to being high in protein, almond milk is an excellent source of vitamin E, an important antioxidant that plays a role in supporting normal heart and brain function, as well as in promoting a healthy complexion.

Nutrients per serving

Calories	69
Fat	2 g
Carbohydrate	14 g
Fiber	3 g
Protein	1 g
Calcium	12 mg
Iron	0.4 mg

• Blender

1 cup	loosely packed baby spinach	250 mL
1 cup	frozen cherries, blueberries or blackberries	250 mL
1 cup	plain almond milk	250 mL

1. In blender, purée spinach, cherries and almond milk until smooth. Pour into two glasses and serve immediately.

Allium Antioxidant

Antioxidant and
antibacterial power!

Nutrients per serving

Calories	165
Fat	0 g
Carbohydrate	41 g
Fiber	6 g
Protein	3 g
Calcium	66 mg
Iron	0.9 mg

- **Blender**

¾ cup	carrot juice	175 mL
1	stalk celery, cut into chunks	1
¼	onion	¼
½	clove garlic	½
1	apple, quartered	1

1. In blender, combine carrot juice, celery, onion, garlic and apple. Secure lid and blend (from low to high if using a variable-speed blender) until smooth.

Appled Beet

Makes 1 serving

Rich in antioxidants
and magnesium.

Nutrients per serving

Calories	225
Fat	1 g
Carbohydrate	56 g
Fiber	9 g
Protein	4 g
Calcium	58 mg
Iron	2.5 mg

- **Blender**

½ cup	apple juice	125 mL
1 cup	cooked sliced beets	250 mL
1	apple, quartered	1
½ cup	packed spinach	125 mL
1 tsp	fresh thyme	5 mL

1. In blender, combine apple juice, beets, apple, spinach and thyme. Secure lid and blend (from low to high if using a variable-speed blender) until smooth.

Brocco-Carrot

Nutrients per serving

Calories	250
Fat	2 g
Carbohydrate	56 g
Fiber	16 g
Protein	11 g
Calcium	368 mg
Iron	5.5 mg

• **Blender**

½ cup	carrot juice	125 mL
¼ cup	apple juice	60 mL
1 cup	cooked fresh or thawed frozen spinach	250 mL
½ cup	chopped cooked or thawed frozen broccoli	125 mL
1	apple, quartered	1
¼ tsp	salt (or to taste)	1 mL

1. In blender, combine carrot juice, apple juice, spinach, broccoli and apple. Secure lid and blend (from low to high if using a variable-speed blender) until smooth. Season with salt. Serve hot or cold with a spoon.

C-Green

Immune-boosting and detoxifying!

Nutrients per serving

Calories	255
Fat	15 g
Carbohydrate	32 g
Fiber	10 g
Protein	4 g
Calcium	52 mg
Iron	2.4 mg

• **Blender**

¾ cup	apple juice	175 mL
1 cup	chopped spinach	250 mL
½	avocado	½
1 tbsp	chopped fresh parsley	15 mL
1 tbsp	chopped watercress	15 mL

1. In blender, combine apple juice, spinach, avocado, parsley and watercress. Secure lid and blend (from low to high if using a variable-speed blender) until smooth.

Popeye's Power

A great builder!

Nutrients per serving	
Calories	143
Fat	0 g
Carbohydrate	33 g
Fiber	6 g
Protein	5 g
Calcium	58 mg
Iron	1.9 mg

• **Blender**

½ cup	beet or carrot juice	125 mL
1 cup	cooked diced beets	250 mL
½ cup	chopped spinach	125 mL
½ cup	cooked chopped carrots	125 mL
1	1 inch (2.5 cm) piece dandelion root, chopped	1
1 tbsp	molasses (optional)	15 mL

1. In blender, combine beet juice, beets, spinach, carrots, dandelion root and molasses (if using). Secure lid and blend (from low to high if using a variable-speed blender) until smooth.

Migraine Tonic

Makes 1 serving

Helps reduce symptoms.

Nutrients per serving	
Calories	65
Fat	0 g
Carbohydrate	15 g
Fiber	2 g
Protein	2 g
Calcium	43 mg
Iron	0.9 mg

• **Blender**

¼ cup	beet juice	60 mL
¼ cup	carrot juice	60 mL
¼ cup	chopped cantaloupe	60 mL
1	stalk celery, cut into chunks	1
1 tbsp	chopped fresh parsley	15 mL
1	½-inch (1 cm) slice gingerroot	1
1 tsp	fresh rosemary	5 mL
¼ tsp	cayenne pepper	1 mL
10	drops feverfew tincture	10

1. In blender, combine beet juice, carrot juice, cantaloupe, celery, parsley, gingerroot, rosemary, cayenne and feverfew tincture. Secure lid and blend (from low to high if using a variable-speed blender) until smooth.

Soups

Vegetable Stock

Here's the perfect stock for all you vegetarians out there. It keeps for up to 6 months if frozen in airtight containers.

Tip

The advantage of making your own stock is that the flavor is richer. As well, there is virtually no sodium compared to commercially prepared bouillon, which contains about 780 mg sodium per 1-cup (250 mL) serving!

6 cups	water	1.5 L
1	large sweet potato, diced	1
2	large celery stalks, chopped	2
2	large leeks, cleaned and sliced	2
1	large onion, chopped	1
½ cup	chopped parsley	125 mL
2	large cloves garlic	2
2	bay leaves	2
¼ tsp	freshly ground black pepper	1 mL
⅛ tsp	salt	0.5 mL

1. In a saucepan, over medium-high heat, combine water, potato, celery, leeks, onion, parsley, garlic, bay leaves, pepper and salt; bring to a boil. Reduce heat to low; simmer, covered, for 1½ hours.

2. Pour mixture through a strainer; discard solids. Refrigerate stock until cold. Stock can be kept, refrigerated, for up to 3 days or frozen in an airtight container.

Nutrients per 1 cup (250 mL)

Calories	41
Fat	0 g
Carbohydrate	9 g
Fiber	2 g
Protein	1 g
Calcium	36 mg
Iron	0.8 mg

Chicken Stock

This nourishing base can be used in many recipes — and it's easy to prepare!

Tip

Refrigerate overnight, remove any layers of fat and freeze in airtight containers for later use.

6 cups	water	1.5 L
2	large chicken pieces (breasts or thighs)	2
1	large carrot, peeled and chopped	1
1	medium onion, quartered	1
1	large celery stalk, chopped	1
3	large cloves garlic	3
1/4 tsp	freshly ground black pepper	1 mL
1/8 tsp	salt	0.5 mL
1/2 cup	chopped parsley	125 mL
2	bay leaves	2

1. In a saucepan, over medium-high heat, combine water, chicken pieces, carrot, onion, celery, garlic, pepper, salt, parsley and bay leaves. Bring to a boil, skimming any foam that rises to the top. Cover, reduce heat to low; simmer for $1\frac{1}{2}$ hours.

2. Pour mixture through a strainer; discard solids. Refrigerate stock until cold; skim fat off surface. Stock can be refrigerated for up to 3 days or frozen in an airtight container.

**Nutrients per
1 cup (250 mL)**

Calories	53
Fat	1 g
Carbohydrate	4 g
Fiber	1 g
Protein	7 g
Calcium	27 mg
Iron	0.8 mg

Creamy Broccoli Soup

Rich in nutrients, but low in fat and calories, this creamy broccoli soup is elegant enough for company, but also just right for an easy weeknight supper. The oats may seem like an unusual addition, but they melt away as the soup simmers, making it all the more velvety.

Tip

If using ready-to-use broth for this recipe, make sure to purchase one that is gluten-free.

• **Food processor, blender or immersion blender**

1 tbsp	extra virgin olive oil	15 mL
1½ cups	chopped onions	375 mL
2	cloves garlic, minced	2
2 tsp	dried basil	10 mL
¼ tsp	freshly ground black pepper	1 mL
1½ lbs	broccoli, coarsely chopped (both florets and peeled stems)	750 g
⅓ cup	large-flake (old-fashioned) rolled oats	75 mL
4 cups	Vegetable Stock (page 178) or reduced-sodium ready-to-use vegetable broth	1 L
1½ cups	water	375 mL

1. In a large saucepan, heat oil over medium-high heat. Add onions and cook, stirring, for 5 to 6 minutes or until softened. Add garlic, basil and pepper; cook, stirring, for 30 seconds.

2. Stir in broccoli, oats, stock and water. Bring to a boil. Reduce heat and simmer, stirring occasionally, for 15 to 18 minutes or until broccoli is tender.

3. Working in batches, transfer soup to food processor (or use immersion blender in pot) and purée until smooth. Return soup to pan (if necessary). Warm over medium heat, stirring, for 1 minute.

Nutrients per serving

Calories	173
Fat	8 g
Carbohydrate	22 g
Fiber	8 g
Protein	7 g
Calcium	119 mg
Iron	2.4 mg

Roasted Cauliflower Quinoa Soup

Makes 8 servings

Roasting cauliflower brings out its best by caramelizing its edges and playing up its nuttiness. The nuttiness quotient is increased with the addition of quinoa, while fresh lime juice and cumin add just the right sharp-savory notes.

Tips

When puréeing soup in a food processor or blender, fill the bowl no more than halfway full at a time.

Try using extra virgin olive oil instead of vegetable oil.

Nutrients per serving

Calories	98
Fat	3 g
Carbohydrate	15 g
Fiber	3 g
Protein	4 g
Calcium	41 mg
Iron	1.0 mg

- **Preheat oven to 450°F (230°C)**
- **Large rimmed baking sheet, lined with foil and sprayed with nonstick cooking spray**
- **Food processor, blender or immersion blender**

6 cups	cauliflower florets (about 1 large head)	1.5 L
4 tsp	vegetable oil, divided	20 mL
	Fine sea salt	
2 cups	chopped onions	500 mL
½ cup	quinoa flakes	125 mL
2 tsp	ground cumin	10 mL
6 cups	water	1.5 L
1½ tbsp	freshly squeezed lime juice	22 mL
	Freshly ground black pepper	
⅓ cup	packed fresh cilantro leaves, roughly chopped	75 mL

1. On prepared baking sheet, toss cauliflower with half the oil and 2 tsp (10 mL) salt. Spread in a single layer. Roast in preheated oven for 35 to 45 minutes, stirring occasionally, until golden brown and tender.

2. Meanwhile, in a large pot, heat the remaining oil over medium-high heat. Add onions and cook, stirring, for 6 to 8 minutes or until softened.

3. Stir in roasted cauliflower, quinoa flakes, cumin, 2 tsp (10 mL) salt and water; bring to a boil. Reduce heat and simmer, stirring occasionally, for 20 minutes or until cauliflower is very soft.

4. Working in batches, transfer soup to food processor (or use immersion blender in pot) and purée until smooth. Return soup to pot (if necessary) and whisk in lime juice. Warm over medium heat, stirring, for 1 minute. Season to taste with salt and pepper. Serve sprinkled with cilantro.

Curried Parsnip Soup with Green Peas

Makes 8 servings

Flavorful and elegant, this soup makes a great introduction to a more substantial meal. Served with whole-grain bread, it is also a satisfying lunch. Complete this soup with a drizzle of coconut milk.

Tip

To enhance the Asian flavors and expand the range of nutrients you consume, substitute extra virgin coconut oil for the olive oil. Its flavors blend very well with the others in this recipe.

Nutrients per serving

Calories	146
Fat	6 g
Carbohydrate	22 g
Fiber	4 g
Protein	3 g
Calcium	79 mg
Iron	2.6 mg

- **Large (minimum 5 quart) slow cooker**
- **Mortar and pestle or spice grinder**
- **Food processor, blender or immersion blender**

2 tsp	cumin seeds	10 mL
1 tsp	coriander seeds	5 mL
1 tbsp	olive oil or extra virgin coconut oil	15 mL
2	onions, finely chopped	2
4	cloves garlic, minced	4
½ tsp	cracked black peppercorns	2 mL
1	1-inch (2.5 cm) cinnamon stick	1
1	bay leaf	1
6 cups	Vegetable Stock (page 178), Chicken Stock (page 179) or reduced-sodium ready-to-use vegetable or chicken broth	1.5 L
4 cups	sliced peeled parsnips (about 1 lb/500 g)	1 L
2 tsp	curry powder, dissolved in 4 tsp (20 mL) freshly squeezed lemon juice	10 mL
2 cups	sweet green peas, thawed if frozen	500 mL
⅓ cup	coconut milk	75 mL

1. In a large dry skillet over medium heat, toast cumin and coriander seeds, stirring, until fragrant and cumin seeds just begin to brown, about 3 minutes. Immediately transfer to a mortar or a spice grinder and grind. Set aside.

2. In same skillet, heat oil over medium heat for 30 seconds. Add onions and cook, stirring, until softened, about 3 minutes. Add garlic, peppercorns, cinnamon stick, bay leaf and reserved cumin and coriander and cook, stirring, for 1 minute. Transfer to slow cooker stoneware. Add stock and parsnips and stir well.

Tip

If you are using large parsnips in this recipe, cut away the woody core and discard.

Make Ahead

This dish can be partially prepared before it is cooked. Complete steps 1 and 2. Cover and refrigerate overnight or for up to 2 days. When you're ready to cook, continue with steps 3 and 4.

3. Cover and cook on Low for 6 hours or on High for 3 hours, until parsnips are tender. Discard cinnamon stick and bay leaf.

4. Working in batches, purée soup in food processor. (You can also do this in the stoneware using an immersion blender.) Return to slow cooker stoneware. Add curry powder solution, green peas and coconut. Cover and cook on High for 20 minutes, until peas are tender and milk is heated through.

Black-Eyed Pea, Collard and Quinoa Soup

Also known as cow peas, black-eyed peas are thought to have originated in North Africa, where they have been eaten for centuries. Here, they pack a spicy broth with plenty of folate, while collard greens add vitamin A and onions contribute vitamin C.

Tips

Try using extra virgin olive oil instead of vegetable oil.

If using ready-to-use broth for this recipe, make sure to purchase one that is gluten-free.

Nutrients per serving	
Calories	218
Fat	3 g
Carbohydrate	26 g
Fiber	8 g
Protein	16 g
Calcium	143 mg
Iron	3.6 mg

2 tsp	vegetable oil	10 mL
2 cups	chopped onions	500 mL
1½ cups	chopped carrots	375 mL
1 cup	chopped celery	250 mL
1 tbsp	ground cumin	15 mL
2 tsp	dried thyme	10 mL
¼ tsp	cayenne pepper	1 mL
8 cups	chopped collard greens (tough stems and center ribs removed)	2 L
¾ cup	quinoa, rinsed	175 mL
8 cups	Chicken Stock (page 179), Vegetable Stock (page 178) or reduced-sodium ready-to-use chicken or vegetable broth	2 L
2	cans (each 14 to 19 oz/398 to 540 mL) black-eyed peas, drained and rinsed	2
1 tbsp	red wine vinegar or cider vinegar	15 mL
	Fine sea salt and freshly ground black pepper	

1. In a large pot, heat oil over medium-high heat. Add onions, carrots and celery; cook, stirring, for 6 to 8 minutes or until softened. Add cumin, thyme and cayenne; cook, stirring, for 30 seconds.

2. Stir in collard greens, quinoa and stock; bring to a boil. Reduce heat to low, cover and simmer, stirring occasionally, for 15 minutes. Stir in peas and vinegar; cover and simmer for 5 minutes or until quinoa is tender. Season to taste with salt and black pepper.

Coconut-Spiked Pumpkin Soup with Cumin and Ginger

Makes 6 to 8 servings

Tips

If using ready-to-use broth for this recipe, make sure to purchase one that is gluten-free. You may need to adjust the quantity of salt depending upon the saltiness of the broth you're using.

If you like heat, increase the quantity of cayenne to ½ tsp (2 mL).

Make Ahead

Complete step 1. Cover and refrigerate for up to 2 days. When you're ready to cook, complete the recipe.

Nutrients per serving

Calories	146
Fat	8 g
Carbohydrate	18 g
Fiber	3 g
Protein	3 g
Calcium	71 mg
Iron	2.6 mg

- Medium to large (4 to 6 quart) slow cooker
- Immersion blender, blender or food processor

1 tbsp	olive oil	15 mL
2	onions, finely chopped	2
2	carrots, peeled and diced	2
2	stalks celery, diced	2
4	cloves garlic, minced	4
2 tbsp	minced gingerroot	30 mL
1 tbsp	ground cumin	15 mL
½ tsp	salt	2 mL
½ tsp	cracked black peppercorns	2 mL
5 cups	Vegetable Stock (page 178) or vegetable broth, divided	1.25 L
6 cups	cubed (½ inch/1 cm) peeled pumpkin or orange squash, such as butternut	1.5 L
¼ tsp	cayenne pepper	1 mL
2 tbsp	freshly squeezed lime juice	30 mL
1 cup	coconut milk	250 mL

1. In a skillet, heat oil over medium heat. Add onions, carrots and celery and cook, stirring, until softened, about 7 minutes. Add garlic, ginger, cumin, salt and peppercorns and cook, stirring for 1 minute. Add 1 cup (250 mL) of the stock and bring to a boil. Transfer to slow cooker stoneware.

2. Add remaining 4 cups (1 L) of stock and pumpkin. Cover and cook on Low for 6 hours, until pumpkin is tender. Purée using an immersion blender. (If you don't have an immersion blender, do this in a stand blender or food processor, in batches, and return to stoneware.)

3. In a small bowl, combine cayenne and lime juice, stirring until cayenne dissolves. Add to slow cooker along with coconut milk. Stir well. Cover and cook on High for 15 minutes to meld flavors.

Indian-Spiced Split Pea and Quinoa Soup

Makes 6 servings

This stunning gold and red soup is positively addictive in the cold winter months: stick-to-the-ribs satisfying without being heavy, subtly spiced with coriander and bright with the finishing flavors of ginger, cilantro and yogurt. Each sip will bring the warmth of the Indian sun to mind.

Tips

Dried yellow lentils or green split peas may be used in place of the yellow split peas.

Try using extra virgin olive oil instead of vegetable oil.

Nutrients per serving

Calories	337
Fat	8 g
Carbohydrate	48 g
Fiber	14 g
Protein	21 g
Calcium	153 mg
Iron	2.8 mg

• **Food processor or blender**

Soup

1 tbsp	vegetable oil	15 mL
2 cups	chopped onions	500 mL
1½ cups	chopped carrots	375 mL
2 tsp	ground coriander	10 mL
1 cup	dried yellow split peas, rinsed	250 mL
7 cups	Chicken Stock (page 179), Vegetable Stock (page 178) or reduced-sodium ready-to-use chicken or vegetable broth	1.75 L
⅔ cup	red or white quinoa, rinsed	150 mL
¾ cup	water (approx.)	175 mL
	Fine sea salt and freshly ground black pepper	
1 cup	plain yogurt	250 mL

Chutney

1	1-inch (2.5 cm) piece gingerroot, roughly chopped	1
1 cup	packed fresh cilantro leaves	250 mL
1 tbsp	freshly squeezed lime juice	15 mL
1 tbsp	toasted sesame oil	15 mL

1. *Soup:* In a large pot, heat oil over medium-high heat. Add onions, carrots and coriander; cook, stirring, for 6 to 8 minutes or until vegetables are softened.

2. Stir in peas and stock; bring to a boil. Reduce heat to low, cover and simmer, stirring occasionally, for 20 minutes. Stir in quinoa, cover and simmer for 15 to 20 minutes or until peas and quinoa are tender.

If using ready-to-use broth for this recipe, make sure to purchase one that is gluten-free.

Experiment with using coconut milk instead of yogurt.

Make Ahead

Store the cooled soup in an airtight container in the refrigerator for up to 3 days or in the freezer for up to 6 months. Thaw overnight in the refrigerator or in the microwave using the Defrost function. Warm soup in a medium saucepan over medium-low heat.

3. Transfer 2 cups (500 mL) of the soup solids to food processor. Add water and purée until smooth. Return purée to pot and simmer, uncovered, stirring often, for 5 minutes to blend the flavors, thinning soup with additional water if too thick. Season to taste with salt and pepper.

4. *Chutney:* In clean food processor, combine ginger, cilantro, lime juice and sesame oil; pulse until finely chopped.

5. Serve soup topped with chutney and dollops of yogurt.

Thai-Style Pumpkin Soup

This soup is both versatile and delicious. It has an exotic combination of flavors and works well as a prelude to a meal. If you prefer a more substantial soup, top each serving with cooked shrimp or scallops, or add some brown rice (see variation, below).

Tips

If using ready-to-use broth for this recipe, make sure to purchase one that is gluten-free.

Coconut cream is the thick part of the liquid that accumulates on the top of canned coconut milk. Scoop out the required quantity, then stir the remainder well for use in the soup.

Nutrients per serving

Calories	130
Fat	8 g
Carbohydrate	14 g
Fiber	2 g
Protein	3 g
Calcium	68 mg
Iron	2.3 mg

- **Large (minimum 6 quart) slow cooker**
- **Food processor, blender or immersion blender**

1 tbsp	olive oil or extra virgin coconut oil	15 mL
2	onions, finely chopped	2
4	cloves garlic, minced	4
2 tbsp	minced gingerroot	30 mL
1 tsp	cracked black peppercorns	5 mL
2	stalks lemongrass, trimmed, smashed and cut in half crosswise	2
1 tbsp	cumin seeds, toasted	15 mL
8 cups	cubed peeled pumpkin or other orange squash (2-inch/5 cm cubes)	2 L
6 cups	Vegetable Stock (page 178), Chicken Stock (page 179) or reduced-sodium ready-to-use vegetable or chicken broth	1.5 L
1 cup	coconut milk	250 mL
1 tsp	Thai red curry paste	5 mL
	Finely grated zest and juice of 1 lime	

Optional Garnishes

Toasted pumpkin seeds

Finely chopped cilantro

1. In a skillet, heat oil over medium heat for 30 seconds. Add onions and cook, stirring, until softened, about 3 minutes. Add garlic, gingerroot, peppercorns, lemongrass and toasted cumin and cook, stirring, for 1 minute. Transfer to slow cooker stoneware. Add pumpkin and stock.

2. Cover and cook on Low for 8 hours or on High for 4 hours, until pumpkin is tender. Skim off 1 tbsp (15 mL) of the coconut cream (see tip, at left). In a small bowl, combine with curry paste and blend well. Add to slow cooker along with remaining coconut milk and lime zest and juice. Cover and cook on High until heated through, about 20 minutes. Discard lemongrass.

3. Working in batches, purée soup in a food processor or blender. (You can also do this in the stoneware using an immersion blender.) Ladle into bowls and sprinkle with optional garnishes as desired.

Spinach, Quinoa and Broccoli Bisque

This gorgeous green soup is elegant enough for company, but also just right for an easy weeknight supper with grilled cheese sandwiches alongside. It's so velvety, it's hard to believe there's neither cream nor butter in this soup.

Tips

For best results, use a vegetable peeler to peel the thick outer layer off the broccoli stems before chopping.

If using ready-to-use broth for this recipe, make sure to purchase one that is gluten-free.

Nutrients per serving

Calories	177
Fat	4 g
Carbohydrate	32 g
Fiber	8 g
Protein	8 g
Calcium	139 mg
Iron	3.7 mg

- **Food processor, blender or immersion blender**

1 tbsp	olive oil	15 mL
1½ cups	chopped onions	375 mL
2	cloves garlic, minced	2
2½ tsp	dried basil	12 mL
¼ tsp	freshly ground black pepper	1 mL
1½ lbs	broccoli, coarsely chopped (florets and peeled stems)	750 g
½ cup	quinoa flakes or quinoa flour	125 mL
6 cups	Vegetable Stock (page 178), Chicken Stock (page 179) or reduced-sodium ready-to-use vegetable or chicken broth	1.5 L
1½ cups	water	375 mL
6 cups	packed spinach leaves	1.5 L
	Fine sea salt and freshly ground black pepper	

1. In a large pot, heat oil over medium-high heat. Add onions and cook, stirring, for 5 to 6 minutes or until softened. Add garlic, basil and pepper; cook, stirring, for 30 seconds.

2. Stir in broccoli, quinoa flakes, stock and water; bring to a boil. Reduce heat and simmer, stirring occasionally, for 15 minutes. Stir in spinach and simmer for 3 to 4 minutes or until broccoli is tender.

3. Working in batches, transfer soup to food processor (or use immersion blender in pot) and purée until smooth. Return soup to pot (if necessary). Warm over medium heat, stirring, for 1 minute. Season to taste with salt and pepper.

Curry-Roasted Squash and Apple Soup

This pretty, fragrant soup is wonderful any time of year, but especially in the fall, when squash and apples are plentiful. But what really makes this soup a winner is the flavorful spices, in particular the turmeric and coriander, which are known for their phytochemical content.

Tip

Try using extra virgin olive oil instead of vegetable oil.

- **Preheat oven to 450°F (230°C)**
- **Rimmed baking sheet, ungreased**
- **Immersion blender or blender**

2 tsp	salt	10 mL
1 tsp	ground coriander	5 mL
1 tsp	ground cumin	5 mL
½ tsp	ground turmeric	2 mL
¼ tsp	ground cinnamon	1 mL
¼ tsp	freshly ground black pepper	1 mL
¼ cup	vegetable oil	60 mL
2 tbsp	cider vinegar	30 mL
4	cloves garlic	4
2	tart apples, peeled and chopped	2
1	butternut squash, peeled and cut into ½-inch (1 cm) pieces (about 8 cups/2 L)	1
1	large onion, chopped	1
6 cups	water (approx.)	1.5 L
½ tsp	garam masala, divided	2 mL
	Salt and freshly ground black pepper	

1. In a small bowl, combine salt, coriander, cumin, turmeric, cinnamon, pepper, oil and vinegar.

2. On baking sheet, combine garlic, apples, squash and onion. Drizzle with spice mixture and toss to coat evenly. Roast in preheated oven, stirring twice, for about 45 minutes or until softened and golden brown.

3. Transfer roasted vegetables to a large pot. Add water and bring to a boil over medium-high heat. Reduce heat and simmer, stirring occasionally, until vegetables are very soft and liquid is reduced by about one-third, about 30 minutes. Remove from heat.

Nutrients per serving

Calories	155
Fat	7 g
Carbohydrate	24 g
Fiber	4 g
Protein	2 g
Calcium	84 mg
Iron	1.3 mg

The soup can be made ahead, cooled, covered and refrigerated for up to 2 days or frozen for up to 2 months (thaw overnight in the refrigerator). Reheat over medium heat until steaming and season to taste before serving.

4. Using an immersion blender in pot (or transferring soup in batches to an upright blender), purée until very smooth. Return to pot, if necessary.

5. Reheat over medium heat until steaming, stirring often. Thin with a little water, if necessary, to desired consistency. Stir in half the garam masala and season to taste with salt and pepper. Ladle into warmed bowls and serve sprinkled with remaining garam masala.

Variation

Replace squash with 2 large sweet potatoes, peeled and cut into ½-inch (1 cm) pieces.

Swiss Chard, Sweet Potato and Quinoa Soup

Here, the distinctive, mellow sweetness of sweet potatoes is augmented by the subtle sesame flavor of quinoa and the grassy flavor of Swiss chard for a harmonious balance of flavors and textures.

Tip

If using ready-to-use broth for this recipe, make sure to purchase one that is gluten-free.

2 tsp	extra virgin olive oil	10 mL
2 cups	chopped onions	500 mL
2	large sweet potatoes (each about 1 lb/500 g), peeled and cut into ¼-inch (0.5 cm) cubes	2
¾ cup	quinoa, rinsed	175 mL
	Freshly ground black pepper	
5 cups	Chicken Stock (page 179), Vegetable Stock (page 178) or reduced-sodium ready-to-use chicken or vegetable broth	1.25 L
6 cups	packed chopped Swiss chard, tough stems removed	1.5 L
2 tbsp	freshly squeezed lemon juice	30 mL
	Fine sea salt	
½ cup	basil pesto (store-bought or page 215)	125 mL

1. In a large pot, heat oil over medium-high heat. Add onions and cook, stirring, for 5 to 6 minutes or until softened.

2. Stir in sweet potatoes, quinoa, ¾ tsp (3 mL) pepper and stock; bring to a boil. Reduce heat to low, cover, leaving lid ajar, and simmer, stirring occasionally, for 20 to 25 minutes or until sweet potatoes are very tender but not falling apart.

3. Stir in Swiss chard, cover and simmer for 5 minutes or until greens are wilted. Stir in lemon juice. Season to taste with salt and pepper.

4. Serve each bowl of soup with a dollop of pesto swirled in.

Nutrients per serving

Calories	334
Fat	14 g
Carbohydrate	40 g
Fiber	6 g
Protein	14 g
Calcium	145 mg
Iron	3.5 mg

Lentil and Spinach Soup

This nourishing soup provides iron and calcium and is high in protein and fiber.

Tips

Look for bags of spinach that have been frozen in small cubes rather than in a large block. You can measure the cubes and add them to the pot without thawing them. If you can't find them, use ½ cup (125 mL) drained thawed chopped spinach.

If using ready-to-use broth for this recipe, make sure to purchase one that is gluten-free.

2 tbsp	olive oil	30 mL
2	cloves garlic, minced	2
¼ cup	chopped onion	60 mL
¼ cup	chopped celery	60 mL
½ cup	chopped carrots	125 mL
2 cups	rinsed drained canned lentils	500 mL
1 cup	frozen spinach cubes	250 mL
4 cups	Chicken Stock (page 179), Vegetable Stock (page 178) or reduced-sodium ready-to-use chicken or vegetable broth	1 L
	Salt and freshly ground black pepper	

1. In a large saucepan, heat oil over medium heat. Sauté garlic, onion, celery and carrots for 3 to 4 minutes or until softened.

2. Stir in lentils, spinach and stock; bring to a boil over high heat. Cover, leaving lid ajar, reduce heat to low and simmer, stirring occasionally, for 30 minutes or until vegetables are tender (or for up to 1 hour if you prefer a very soft texture). Season to taste with salt and pepper.

Nutrients per serving

Calories	220
Fat	8 g
Carbohydrate	26 g
Fiber	10 g
Protein	13 g
Calcium	81 mg
Iron	5.0 mg

Lemony Lentil Soup with Spinach

This soup is so light and refreshing, it's hard to believe that it's also packed with nutrition.

Tips

Try using extra virgin olive oil instead of vegetable oil.

If your stock is unsalted, add 1 tsp (5 mL) salt (or to taste) with the stock.

If using ready-to-use broth for this recipe, make sure to purchase one that is gluten-free.

1 tbsp	vegetable oil	15 mL
1 cup	diced onion	250 mL
1 tbsp	minced garlic	15 mL
Pinch	cayenne pepper	Pinch
	Freshly ground black pepper	
1	package (10 oz/300 g) frozen chopped spinach or 1 bag (10 oz/300 g) fresh spinach, stems removed and chopped	1
1	can (19 oz/540 mL) lentils, drained and rinsed	1
5 cups	Vegetable Stock (page 178), Chicken Stock (page 179) or reduced-sodium ready-to-use vegetable or chicken broth	1.25 L
¼ cup	freshly squeezed lemon juice	60 mL
	Salt	

1. In a large saucepan, heat oil over medium heat. Add onion and cook, stirring, until softened, about 3 minutes. Add garlic, cayenne and black pepper to taste. Cook, stirring, for 1 minute.

2. Add spinach and cook, stirring and breaking up with spoon, until thawed (if frozen) or wilted (if fresh). Add lentils and stock. Bring to a boil. Reduce heat to low and simmer for 15 minutes to cook spinach and combine flavors. Stir in lemon juice, and salt to taste. Serve immediately.

Variation

Curried Lentil and Spinach Soup: Add 1 to 3 tsp (5 to 15 mL) curry powder, depending upon the degree of spice you prefer, with the garlic.

Nutrients per serving

Calories	215
Fat	4 g
Carbohydrate	36 g
Fiber	16 g
Protein	12 g
Calcium	131 mg
Iron	1.8 mg

Easy Chicken Quinoa Soup

Makes 6 servings

An old-fashioned, ever-comforting favorite gets a newfangled twist, thanks to quinoa in place of the usual noodles or rice.

Tip

If using ready-to-use broth for this recipe, make sure to purchase one that is gluten-free.

Make Ahead

Store the cooled soup in an airtight container in the refrigerator for up to 3 days or in the freezer for up to 6 months. Thaw overnight in the refrigerator or in the microwave using the Defrost function. Warm soup in a medium saucepan over medium-low heat.

Nutrients per serving	
Calories	194
Fat	4 g
Carbohydrate	28 g
Fiber	4 g
Protein	12 g
Calcium	64 mg
Iron	2.5 mg

2 tsp	olive oil	10 mL
1 cup	chopped onions	250 mL
1 cup	chopped carrots	250 mL
1 cup	chopped celery	250 mL
½ tsp	freshly ground black pepper	2 mL
1 cup	quinoa, rinsed	250 mL
6 cups	Chicken Stock (page 179), Vegetable Stock (page 178) or reduced-sodium ready-to-use chicken or vegetable broth	1.5 L
2 cups	diced or shredded cooked chicken breast	500 mL
	Fine sea salt and freshly ground black pepper	
3 tbsp	chopped fresh flat-leaf (Italian) parsley	45 mL

1. In a large pot, heat oil over medium-high heat. Add onions, carrots, celery and pepper; cook, stirring, for 6 to 8 minutes or until vegetables are softened.

2. Stir in quinoa and stock; bring to a boil. Reduce heat to low, cover and simmer, stirring occasionally, for 15 to 20 minutes or until quinoa is tender.

3. Stir in chicken. Simmer, uncovered, for 5 minutes to heat through and blend the flavors. Season to taste with salt and pepper. Serve sprinkled with parsley.

Gingery Chicken and Wild Rice Soup

Makes 6 servings

The addition of a flavorful whole grain, leeks and a hint of ginger is a particularly delicious spin on classic chicken and rice soup. Make the stock a day ahead so it can be refrigerated, which makes easy work of skimming off the fat (see tip, opposite). This makes a great light dinner accompanied by whole-grain rolls and a tossed salad.

1	whole chicken (about 3 lbs/1.5 kg), cut into pieces	1
1	onion, coarsely chopped	1
2	carrots, peeled and diced	2
2	stalks celery, diced	2
4	sprigs parsley	4
1	clove garlic	1
1	bay leaf	1
½ tsp	salt	2 mL
½ tsp	cracked black peppercorns	2 mL
12 cups	water	3 L
1 tbsp	olive oil	15 mL
2	large leeks, white part only, cleaned and sliced	2
2	cloves garlic, minced	2
2 tbsp	minced gingerroot	30 mL
1 cup	brown and wild rice mixture, rinsed and drained	250 mL

1. In a stockpot, combine chicken, onion, carrots, celery, parsley, whole garlic, bay leaf, salt, peppercorns and water. Bring to a boil over high heat. Using a slotted spoon, skim off foam. Reduce heat to medium-low and simmer, uncovered, until chicken is falling off the bone, about 1½ hours. Drain, reserving chicken and liquid separately. Let cool. Cut the chicken into bite-size pieces, discarding skin and bones. Skim off fat from the stock (see tip, at right).

2. Measure 2 cups (500 mL) of chicken and set aside in the refrigerator. (Refrigerate the remainder for other uses.)

Nutrients per serving

Calories	269
Fat	8 g
Carbohydrate	27 g
Fiber	2 g
Protein	22 g
Calcium	51 mg
Iron	1.9 mg

3. In a large saucepan or stockpot, heat oil over medium heat for 30 seconds. Add leeks and cook, stirring, until softened, about 5 minutes. Add minced garlic and ginger and cook, stirring, for 1 minute. Add rice and toss to coat. Add reserved stock and bring to a boil. Reduce heat and simmer, uncovered, until rice is quite tender, about 1 hour. Add reserved chicken. Cover and simmer until chicken is heated through, about 15 minutes.

Variation

Substitute an equal quantity of rinsed wild rice for the mixture. You may need to increase the cooking time, depending upon the size of the grains.

Turkey Wild Rice Soup

Makes 8 to 10 servings

Here's a low-sodium turkey soup recipe for the slow cooker. As the wonderful aromas start to fill the kitchen, you'll say, "It smells like turkey dinner!"

Tips

Try using extra virgin olive oil instead of canola oil.

If using ready-to-use broth for this recipe, make sure to purchase one that is gluten-free.

Nutrients per serving

Calories	125
Fat	5 g
Carbohydrate	10 g
Fiber	1 g
Protein	11 g
Calcium	31 mg
Iron	1.1 mg

• **Medium to large (minimum 4 quart) slow cooker**

2 tsp	canola oil	10 mL
1 lb	lean ground turkey	500 g
1	clove garlic, minced	1
1 cup	coarsely chopped onion	250 mL
1 cup	coarsely chopped celery	250 mL
1 cup	coarsely chopped carrots	250 mL
½ cup	wild rice	125 mL
4 cups	Chicken Stock (page 179) or reduced-sodium ready-to-use chicken broth	1 L
½ tsp	dried sage	2 mL
½ tsp	dried savory	2 mL
½ tsp	dried thyme	2 mL
½ tsp	dried marjoram	2 mL
½ tsp	freshly ground black pepper	2 mL
½ tsp	salt (optional)	2 mL
2 to 3 tbsp	chopped fresh parsley	30 to 45 mL

1. In a large nonstick skillet, heat oil over medium heat. Brown turkey, breaking it up with a spoon, for about 8 minutes or until no longer pink. Drain off excess fat.

2. Transfer turkey to slow cooker stoneware and stir in garlic, onion, celery, carrots, wild rice, stock, 2 cups (500 mL) water, sage, savory, thyme, marjoram, pepper and salt (if using). Cover and cook on High for 4 to 5 hours or until vegetables and rice are tender. Ladle into bowls and garnish with parsley to taste.

Variation

Use long-grain brown rice instead of wild rice.

This recipe courtesy of Dorraine Hayward.

Salads and Dressings

Wilted Spinach Salad

This simple salad is a wonderful dish that can be served on its own or used as a base for nutritious toppings such as guacamole or hummus.

Tips

If you use baby spinach to make this recipe, use twice as much because it is lighter and less dense.

You may replace the lemon juice with an equal quantity of lime juice.

6 cups	chopped spinach leaves (see tip, at left)	1.5 L
½ cup	extra virgin olive oil	125 mL
¼ cup	freshly squeezed lemon juice	60 mL
1 tsp	fine sea salt	5 mL

1. In a bowl, toss together spinach, olive oil, lemon juice and salt until well combined. Set aside for 15 minutes, until spinach wilts. Serve immediately or transfer to an airtight container and refrigerate for up to 2 days.

Nutrients per serving

Calories	517
Fat	56 g
Carbohydrate	10 g
Fiber	4 g
Protein	2 g
Calcium	53 mg
Iron	2.3 mg

Simple Marinated Kale Salad

This is an easy way to marinate kale, which is often called a "superfood."

Tips

Before chopping the kale, remove the long stem that runs up through the leaf. Use only the leafy green parts.

Cut the kale very thinly, to expose as much surface area as possible to the marinade.

For a quick hit of protein, sprinkle some hemp seeds overtop.

2 cups	thinly sliced kale (see tips, at left)	500 mL
1/4 cup	extra virgin olive oil	60 mL
2 tbsp	freshly squeezed lemon juice	30 mL
1 tsp	fine sea salt	5 mL

1. In a bowl, toss together kale, olive oil, lemon juice and salt. Set aside for 10 minutes to soften. Serve immediately or transfer to an airtight container and refrigerate for up to 3 days. Before serving, toss with dressing, if desired.

Variation

Substitute 1/4 cup (60 mL) flax oil for the olive oil and 2 tsp (10 mL) apple cider vinegar for the lemon juice.

Nutrients per serving

Calories	277
Fat	29 g
Carbohydrate	8 g
Fiber	2 g
Protein	2 g
Calcium	91 mg
Iron	1.2 mg

Mega-Green Hemp Bowl

Makes 2 servings

Here's an easy way to add nutritious green vegetables to your diet. This salad takes very little time to prepare and for convenience can be made ahead and refrigerated for up to 2 days.

Tips

Before chopping the kale, remove the long stem that runs up through the leaf almost to the top. Use only the leafy green parts.

Dark leafy greens, such as kale and Swiss chard, contain appreciable amounts of calcium and magnesium.

2 cups	chopped spinach leaves	500 mL
1 cup	thinly sliced kale (see tip, at left)	250 mL
1 cup	thinly sliced chard	250 mL
½ cup	arugula	125 mL
3 tbsp	raw shelled hemp seeds	45 mL
½ cup	hemp oil	125 mL
¼ cup	freshly squeezed lemon juice	60 mL
1 tsp	fine sea salt	5 mL

1. In a bowl, toss spinach, kale, chard, arugula and hemp seeds. Add hemp oil, lemon juice and salt and toss well. Set aside for 15 minutes to soften the greens. Serve immediately or transfer to an airtight container and refrigerate for up to 2 days.

Nutrients per serving

Calories	524
Fat	62 g
Carbohydrate	11 g
Fiber	2 g
Protein	7 g
Calcium	91 mg
Iron	3.6 mg

Carrot and Ginger Salad

Makes 4 servings

This salad is brightly colored and full of flavor. As a bonus, carrots are an excellent source of beta carotene, which becomes vitamin A in the body.

Tips

For added convenience, shredded carrots can be purchased at the grocery store.

To peel gingerroot without a vegetable peeler, use the edge of a large spoon to scrape the skin off.

Gingerroot can be grated ahead of time and frozen in 1-tbsp (15 mL) portions, ready for use.

Nutrients per serving	
Calories	122
Fat	9 g
Carbohydrate	12 g
Fiber	4 g
Protein	2 g
Calcium	71 mg
Iron	0.6 mg

• Food processor

1 lb	carrots, cut into 3-inch (7.5 cm) lengths	500 g
2 tbsp	extra virgin olive oil	30 mL
1 tbsp	freshly grated gingerroot	15 mL
1 tbsp	poppy seeds	15 mL
	Salt and freshly ground black pepper	

1. In food processor fitted with shredding blade, shred carrots. Transfer to a large salad bowl. Add oil, ginger, poppy seeds, and salt and pepper to taste. Cover and refrigerate to allow flavors to meld, about 30 minutes. Serve at room temperature.

Jicama, Carrot and Ginger Salad

Fresh and oil free, this super-healthy salad brings color and zest to any table.

Tip

To garner orange flesh, slice off both ends of orange. Use a sharp paring knife to remove the peel and pith. Slice into the orange along separating membrane and remove segments.

	Grated zest and juice of 2 limes	
½ tsp	cayenne pepper	2 mL
½ tsp	salt	2 mL
½	large jicama, peeled and cut into matchsticks	½
3	large carrots, peeled and grated	3
1	1-inch (2.5 cm) piece gingerroot, cut into thin matchsticks	1
2	navel oranges, peeled and cut into segments (see tip, at left)	2

1. In a small bowl, whisk together lime zest, lime juice, cayenne pepper and salt.
2. In a large bowl, toss together jicama, carrots and ginger. Pour lime mixture over salad and toss to coat. Gently fold in orange segments. Taste and adjust seasonings and serve.

Nutrients per serving

Calories	78
Fat	0 g
Carbohydrate	19 g
Fiber	7 g
Protein	2 g
Calcium	46 mg
Iron	0.8 mg

Avocado and Cucumber Salad

This light and creamy side salad will play games with your taste buds. Serve over crisp romaine lettuce leaves or baby spinach.

Tip

Do not chop the parsley too finely for this recipe. You want it to be a main ingredient in this salad, as opposed to a side note. Similarly, by keeping the avocado and cucumber chunky, you ensure a salad-like result. If the ingredients were diced it would be more like a salsa.

2 cups	cubed avocado (about 3 medium, cut into 1-inch/2.5 cm cubes)	500 mL
1 cup	cubed seeded peeled cucumber (about ½ large, cut into 1-inch/2.5 cm cubes)	250 mL
⅓ cup	coarsely chopped flat-leaf (Italian) parsley leaves	75 mL
3 tbsp	flax oil	45 mL
2 tbsp	freshly squeezed lemon or lime juice	30 mL
1½ tsp	fine sea salt	7 mL
Pinch	freshly ground black pepper	Pinch

1. In a serving bowl, toss avocado, cucumber, parsley, flax oil, lemon juice, salt and freshly ground pepper until well coated. Serve immediately.

Variations

Add ½ cup (125 mL) chopped tomatoes.

Replace the parsley with an equal quantity of coarsely chopped cilantro leaves and add 1 tsp (5 mL) chili powder and ½ tsp (2 mL) ground cumin to give this salad a Southwestern spin.

Nutrients per serving

Calories	218
Fat	21 g
Carbohydrate	8 g
Fiber	6 g
Protein	2 g
Calcium	21 mg
Iron	0.8 mg

Autumn Harvest Salad and Harvest Dressing

An abundance of delicious root vegetables makes for a nutrient-packed salad. Using a food processor to shred the vegetables makes it quick and easy too!

Tip

Shaving or shredding the root vegetables makes them easy to combine and digest.

1 cup	shredded carrot	250 mL
½ cup	shredded turnip	125 mL
½ cup	shredded beet	125 mL
1	apple, diced	1
2	green onions, thinly sliced on the diagonal	2
2 tbsp	fresh thyme leaves	30 mL
1 tbsp	chopped fresh sage	15 mL
⅓ cup	Harvest Dressing (see recipe, opposite)	75 mL
¼ cup	coarsely chopped cashews	60 mL
3 tbsp	sesame seeds	45 mL

1. In a large salad bowl, combine carrot, turnip, beet, apple, green onions, thyme and sage. Toss well to combine. Drizzle Harvest Dressing over top and toss well. Scatter cashew nuts and sesame seeds over top and serve immediately.

Nutrients per serving

Calories	228
Fat	18 g
Carbohydrate	17 g
Fiber	5 g
Protein	5 g
Calcium	69 mg
Iron	2.0 mg

Harvest Dressing

Here's a great change-of-season recipe — the perfect dressing to accompany a hearty autumn salad.

Tip

Any finely shredded herb or leaf vegetable is called "chiffonade."

1	whole head garlic, roasted (or 1 clove garlic, finely chopped)	1
3 tbsp	olive oil	45 mL
1 tbsp	tamari	15 mL
1 tbsp	freshly squeezed lemon juice	15 mL
2 tbsp	chiffonade basil (see tip, at left)	30 mL
	Salt (optional)	

1. In a jar with lid or a small bowl, combine garlic, oil, tamari, lemon juice and basil. (If using roasted garlic, squeeze soft cloves into the container and mash with a fork.) Shake or whisk ingredients to mix well. Taste and adjust seasonings, adding salt if needed.

**Nutrients
per 1 tbsp (15 mL)**

Calories	76
Fat	8 g
Carbohydrate	1 g
Fiber	0 g
Protein	1 g
Calcium	4 mg
Iron	0.1 mg

Avocado, Grapefruit and Quinoa Salad

Pretty in shades of pink and green, plus the polka-dot accents of poppy seeds, this easy salad is refreshing and satisfying at the same time. The quinoa and avocados give the salad real substance, and the grapefruit, mustard and red onion provide zest.

Tip

Avocados come in several varieties, but Hass are the most widely available. A Hass avocado — notable for its dark, bumpy skin and rich, buttery flesh — is ideal in this simple salad, but any other variety may be used in its place.

Nutrients per serving	
Calories	340
Fat	20 g
Carbohydrate	39 g
Fiber	9 g
Protein	7 g
Calcium	65 mg
Iron	2.2 mg

2	large ruby red grapefruits	2
1 tsp	ground cumin	5 mL
3 tbsp	extra virgin olive oil	45 mL
1 tbsp	agave nectar or liquid honey	15 mL
2 tsp	Dijon mustard	10 mL
3 cups	cooked quinoa, cooled	750 mL
2	small firm-ripe Hass avocados, diced	2
1/3 cup	finely chopped red onion	75 mL
2 tbsp	chopped fresh mint	30 mL
	Fine sea salt and freshly cracked black pepper	
1 tbsp	poppy seeds	15 mL

1. Using a sharp knife, cut peel and pith from grapefruits. Working over a small bowl, cut between membranes to release segments. Squeeze the membranes to release any remaining juice into the bowl. Remove segments and coarsely chop.

2. To the grapefruit juice, whisk in cumin, oil, agave nectar and mustard.

3. In a large bowl, combine grapefruit segments, quinoa, avocados, red onion and mint. Add dressing and gently toss to coat. Season to taste with salt and pepper. Cover and refrigerate for at least 30 minutes, until chilled, or for up to 2 hours.

4. Just before serving, sprinkle with poppy seeds.

Pomegranate and Quinoa Salad with Sunflower Seeds

This sensational combination of pomegranates, quinoa and sunflower seeds is worth making again and again.

Tip

To remove pomegranate seeds, score the fruit around the circumference and place it in a large bowl of water. Break the pomegranate open underwater to free the white seed sacs. The seeds will sink to the bottom of the bowl, and the membrane will float to the top. Strain out the seeds and put them in a separate bowl.

1 cup	quinoa, rinsed	250 mL
2 cups	water	500 mL
2 tsp	finely grated lemon zest	10 mL
2 tbsp	freshly squeezed lemon juice	30 mL
2 tbsp	extra virgin olive oil	30 mL
1 tbsp	agave nectar or liquid honey	15 mL
½ tsp	fine sea salt	2 mL
¾ cup	pomegranate seeds	175 mL
⅓ cup	lightly salted roasted sunflower seeds	75 mL
¼ cup	packed fresh mint leaves, chopped	60 mL
¼ cup	packed fresh cilantro leaves, chopped	60 mL

1. In a medium saucepan, combine quinoa and water. Bring to a boil over medium-high heat. Reduce heat to low, cover and simmer for 15 to 18 minutes or until water is absorbed. Transfer to a large bowl and let cool completely.

2. In a small bowl, whisk together lemon zest, lemon juice, oil, agave nectar and salt.

3. To the quinoa, add pomegranate seeds, sunflower seeds, mint and cilantro. Add dressing and gently toss to coat.

Variation

An equal amount of dried cranberries or chopped dried cherries may be used in place of the pomegranate seeds.

Nutrients per serving	
Calories	227
Fat	11 g
Carbohydrate	27 g
Fiber	4 g
Protein	6 g
Calcium	25 mg
Iron	2.8 mg

Lemony Brussels Sprouts Quinoa Salad

Makes 6 servings

When Brussels sprouts are lightly cooked — as they are in this simple yet vibrant salad — and then complemented with assertive flavors, such as tart lemon and nutty quinoa, their intense flavor is beautifully balanced.

Tip

Trim the root end from Brussels sprouts and cut off any loose, thick outer leaves, then rinse well to remove any grit that may have gathered under loose leaves.

Nutrients per serving

Calories	228
Fat	12 g
Carbohydrate	28 g
Fiber	5 g
Protein	7 g
Calcium	51 mg
Iron	2.2 mg

- Steamer basket

1 lb	Brussels sprouts, trimmed	500 g
	Ice water	
1 tsp	finely grated lemon zest	5 mL
2 tbsp	freshly squeezed lemon juice	30 mL
2 tbsp	extra virgin olive oil	30 mL
2 tbsp	liquid honey	30 mL
1 tbsp	whole-grain Dijon mustard	15 mL
2 cups	cooked red, black or white quinoa, cooled	500 mL
	Fine sea salt and freshly cracked black pepper	
½ cup	chopped toasted walnuts	125 mL

1. Place Brussels sprouts in a steamer basket set over a large saucepan of boiling water. Cover and steam for 5 to 6 minutes or until tender-crisp but still bright green. Transfer to a large bowl of ice water to stop the cooking. Drain and pat dry with paper towels. Using a very sharp knife or a mandolin, thinly slice Brussels sprouts lengthwise.

2. In a small bowl, whisk together lemon zest, lemon juice, oil, honey and mustard.

3. In a large bowl, combine Brussels sprouts and quinoa. Add dressing and gently toss to coat. Season to taste with salt and pepper. Cover and refrigerate for at least 30 minutes, until chilled, or for up to 2 hours.

4. Just before serving, sprinkle with walnuts.

Herbed Chicken and Pomegranate Salad

This stellar salad relies on varied tastes and textures — nutty quinoa, succulent roast chicken, aromatic fresh herbs, tart, crunchy pomegranate seeds and rich, slightly sweet pine nuts — to impress one and all.

3 cups	cooked quinoa, cooled	750 mL
2 cups	shredded rotisserie, grilled or poached chicken breast	500 mL
1 cup	pomegranate seeds (see tip, page 211)	250 mL
2 tsp	finely grated lime zest	10 mL
2 tbsp	freshly squeezed lime juice	30 mL
2 tbsp	extra virgin olive oil	30 mL
1 tbsp	liquid honey	15 mL
	Fine sea salt and freshly cracked black pepper	
¼ cup	packed fresh mint leaves, chopped	60 mL
¼ cup	packed fresh cilantro leaves, chopped	60 mL
⅓ cup	toasted pine nuts or sliced almonds	75 mL

1. In a large bowl, combine quinoa, chicken and pomegranate seeds.

2. In a small bowl, whisk together lime zest, lime juice, oil and honey. Add to quinoa mixture and gently toss to coat. Season to taste with salt and pepper. Cover and refrigerate for at least 30 minutes, until chilled, or for up to 4 hours.

3. Just before serving, add mint and cilantro, gently tossing to combine. Sprinkle with pine nuts.

Variation

An equal amount of dried cranberries or chopped dried cherries may be used in place of the pomegranate seeds.

Nutrients per serving	
Calories	439
Fat	19 g
Carbohydrate	45 g
Fiber	6 g
Protein	24 g
Calcium	35 mg
Iron	3.8 mg

Lemon Vinaigrette

⅓ cup	extra virgin olive oil	75 mL
3 tbsp	freshly squeezed lemon juice	45 mL
2 tbsp	chopped fresh dill	30 mL
	Salt and freshly ground black pepper	

1. In a container with a tight-fitting lid, combine oil, lemon juice and dill. Cover and shake well to blend. Season to taste with salt and pepper.

Nutrients per 1 tbsp (15 mL)

Calories	79
Fat	9 g
Carbohydrate	1 g
Fiber	0 g
Protein	0 g
Calcium	14 mg
Iron	0.4 mg

Detox Vinaigrette

• **Blender**

¾ cup	flax oil	175 mL
½ tsp	finely grated lemon zest	2 mL
¼ cup	freshly squeezed lemon juice	60 mL
2 tsp	chopped gingerroot	10 mL
½ tsp	dried dulse flakes	2 mL
¼ tsp	fine sea salt	1 mL
Pinch	cayenne pepper	Pinch

1. In blender, combine flax oil, lemon zest, lemon juice, ginger, dulse, salt and cayenne. Blend at high speed until smooth. Serve immediately or cover and refrigerate for up to 5 days.

Variation

This dressing has a fairly strong lemon flavor. If you prefer a more neutral taste, add ¼ cup (60 mL) extra virgin olive oil and 2 tbsp (30 mL) agave nectar.

Nutrients per 1 tbsp (15 mL)

Calories	58
Fat	7 g
Carbohydrate	0 g
Fiber	0 g
Protein	0 g
Calcium	0 mg
Iron	0.0 mg

Basil Pesto Sauce

**Makes about
2 cups (500 mL)**

Nutrients per 1 tbsp (15 mL)	
Calories	26
Fat	3 g
Carbohydrate	1 g
Fiber	0 g
Protein	0 g
Calcium	9 mg
Iron	0.2 mg

• **Food processor or blender**

3 cups	packed fresh basil leaves	750 mL
2	cloves garlic	2
1/3 cup	extra virgin olive oil	75 mL
1/3 cup	slivered almonds or pine nuts	75 mL

1. In food processor, process basil, garlic, oil and almonds until coarsely chopped. Process until well combined.

Variation

Pesto Vinaigrette Dressing: Combine 1/3 cup (75 mL) olive oil, 2 tbsp (30 mL) white wine vinegar and 1 tbsp (15 mL) Basil Pesto Sauce.

Basil, Spinach and Walnut Pesto

**Makes about
2 cups (500 mL)**

Nutrients per 1 tbsp (15 mL)	
Calories	27
Fat	3 g
Carbohydrate	1 g
Fiber	1 g
Protein	1 g
Calcium	6 mg
Iron	0.2 mg

• **Food processor**

1/4 cup	freshly squeezed lemon juice	60 mL
3	cloves garlic	3
2 tsp	fine sea salt	10 mL
1 tsp	freshly ground black pepper	5 mL
1 cup	fresh basil leaves	250 mL
4 cups	chopped spinach leaves	1 L
1/2 cup	chopped walnut halves or pieces	125 mL
1/4 cup	flax oil	60 mL

1. In food processor, process lemon juice, garlic, salt and pepper until no large pieces of garlic remain. Add basil, spinach and walnuts and process until smooth. With the motor running, gradually add flax oil through the feed tube until blended.

2. Transfer to a bowl and serve immediately or cover and refrigerate for up to 3 days.

Cashew Sour Cream

You will be surprised at how creamy and rich this non-dairy version of sour cream is. It is a perfect finish for many recipes in this book.

Tips

To soak the cashews for this recipe, cover with 4 cups (1 L) water. Set aside for 30 minutes. Drain, discarding soaking water. Rinse under cold running water until water runs clear.

Cider vinegar is a healthy addition to your diet. Be sure to use versions containing the "mother." Because they are fermented, they add healthy bacteria to your gut.

Nutrients per 1 tbsp (15 mL)

Calories	29
Fat	2 g
Carbohydrate	2 g
Fiber	0 g
Protein	1 g
Calcium	2 mg
Iron	0.4 mg

● **Blender (preferably high-powered)**

2 cups	raw cashews, soaked (see tip, at left)	500 mL
¾ cup	filtered water	175 mL
⅓ cup	freshly squeezed lemon juice	75 mL
2 tbsp	cider vinegar (see tip, at left)	30 mL
1 tsp	fine sea salt	5 mL

1. In blender, combine soaked cashews, water, lemon juice, vinegar and salt. Blend at high speed until smooth. Transfer to an airtight container and refrigerate for up to 5 days.

Variation

Add 2 tbsp (30 mL) rehydrated sun-dried tomatoes, 1 tsp (5 mL) smoked paprika and ½ tsp (2 mL) chili powder to create a smoky tomato cashew cream.

Fish and Vegetarian Mains

Simple Grilled Fish

This lovely fish dish provides protein, as well as fresh ingredients that contain important nutraceuticals.

Tips

Refrigerate any leftovers in an airtight container for up to 2 days. Flake the fish and mix it with mayonnaise and sliced pickles or tartar sauce to make a sandwich filling.

White fish has a mild flavor and aroma. While pink fish, such as trout, is stronger, it is also higher in beneficial omega-3 fats.

- **Preheat broiler**
- **Rimmed baking sheet, lightly greased**

1 tbsp	chopped fresh parsley	15 mL
1 tbsp	olive oil	15 mL
	Juice of 1 lemon	
4	orange roughy or rainbow trout fillets (about 1¾ lbs/875 g total)	4

1. In a small bowl, combine parsley, oil and lemon juice.
2. Place fish fillets on prepared baking sheet and baste both sides with parsley mixture.
3. Broil for 5 to 10 minutes or until fish is opaque and flakes easily with a fork.

Variation

Substitute tilapia, sole, haddock or halibut for the orange roughy.

This recipe courtesy of Eileen Campbell.

Nutrients per serving

Calories	170
Fat	4 g
Carbohydrate	1 g
Fiber	0 g
Protein	30 g
Calcium	22 mg
Iron	2.3 mg

Black Cod with Fresh Herb Sauce

Firm, meaty black cod fillets stand up beautifully to a fresh sauce fragrant with herbs.

Tips

An equal amount of chopped green onions (green parts only) may be used in place of the chives.

Sea bass, halibut, cod or any other firm white fish fillets may be used in place of the black cod.

If using ready-to-use broth for this recipe, make sure to purchase one that is gluten-free.

- Preheat broiler, with rack set 4 to 6 inches (10 to 15 cm) from the heat source
- Blender or food processor
- Broiler pan, sprayed with nonstick cooking spray (preferably olive oil)

½ cup	packed fresh basil leaves	125 mL
½ cup	packed fresh flat-leaf (Italian) parsley leaves	125 mL
3 tbsp	coarsely chopped fresh chives	45 mL
3 tbsp	Vegetable Stock (page 178) or reduced-sodium ready-to-use vegetable broth	45 mL
2 tbsp	freshly squeezed lemon juice	30 mL
5 tsp	extra virgin olive oil, divided	25 mL
4	skin-on black cod (sablefish) fillets (each about 5 oz/150 g and 1 inch/2.5 cm thick)	4
¼ tsp	fine sea salt	1 mL

1. In blender, combine basil, parsley, chives, stock, lemon juice and 3 tsp (15 mL) of the oil; purée until smooth. Set aside.

2. Place fish, skin side down, on prepared pan. Brush with the remaining oil and sprinkle with salt. Broil for 6 to 8 minutes or until fish is opaque and flakes easily when tested with a fork. Serve with sauce spooned over top.

Nutrients per serving

Calories	301
Fat	25 g
Carbohydrate	2 g
Fiber	1 g
Protein	17 g
Calcium	96 mg
Iron	2.3 mg

Cumin-Crusted Halibut Steaks

Cumin seeds contain many phytochemicals that help promote good health and digestion. They make a tasty replacement for bread crumbs.

Tips

Sea bass, halibut, grouper or any dense white fish are all excellent cooked in this interesting crust.

It is preferable to use toasted cumin seeds, as they have more flavor than ground cumin.

- **Preheat oven to 450°F (230°C)**
- **Coffee or spice grinder**

1 tbsp	cumin seeds	15 mL
½ tsp	salt	2 mL
¼ tsp	freshly ground black pepper	1 mL
1 lb	skinless halibut or other fish steaks	500 g
2 tsp	olive oil	10 mL
	Chopped fresh parsley (optional)	

1. In a nonstick skillet over medium heat, toast cumin seeds, stirring, for 2 minutes or until golden. Place seeds, salt and pepper in a coffee or spice grinder. Pulse until finely ground. Rub mixture into both sides of fish.

2. Heat olive oil in a large nonstick skillet over medium-high heat. Add fish, in batches, if necessary, and cook for 2 minutes per side or until browned.

3. Return all fish to skillet and wrap handle with foil. Bake in preheated oven for 5 minutes or until fish is opaque and flakes easily when tested with a fork. Sprinkle with parsley (if using).

Nutrients per serving	
Calories	151
Fat	5 g
Carbohydrate	1 g
Fiber	0 g
Protein	24 g
Calcium	23 mg
Iron	1.3 mg

Halibut with Coconut Lime Sauce

Highly prized for its firm, mild flesh, halibut is well worth the occasional splurge at the fish counter. Here, it heads to the islands in a splendid ginger- and lime-infused coconut sauce.

Tips

Try using extra virgin olive oil instead of vegetable oil.

Sea bass, cod or any other firm white fish fillets may be used in place of the halibut.

- **Preheat oven to 350°F (180°C)**
- **9-inch (23 cm) glass baking dish, sprayed with nonstick cooking spray (preferably olive oil)**

1 tsp	vegetable oil	5 mL
2	cloves garlic, minced	2
1 tbsp	minced gingerroot	15 mL
½ tsp	fine sea salt	2 mL
⅛ tsp	cayenne pepper	0.5 mL
½ cup	light coconut milk	125 mL
1 tsp	grated lime zest	5 mL
2 tbsp	freshly squeezed lime juice	30 mL
4	skinless Pacific halibut fillets (each about 5 oz/150 g)	4
½ cup	packed fresh cilantro leaves, chopped	125 mL

1. In a medium skillet, heat oil over medium heat. Add garlic and ginger; cook, stirring, for 2 minutes. Add salt, cayenne, coconut milk, lime zest and lime juice; reduce heat and simmer, stirring occasionally, for 5 minutes.

2. Place fish in prepared baking dish and spoon coconut sauce over top. Bake in preheated oven for 13 to 16 minutes or until fish is opaque and flakes easily when tested with a fork.

3. Place a fillet on each plate and spoon sauce over top. Sprinkle with cilantro.

Nutrients per serving

Calories	149
Fat	5 g
Carbohydrate	2 g
Fiber	0 g
Protein	24 g
Calcium	16 mg
Iron	0.3 mg

Fish for the Sole

Makes 3 servings

Comfort food for the soul — and it does your body good, too!

Nutrients per serving

Calories	220
Fat	10 g
Carbohydrate	8 g
Fiber	1 g
Protein	23 g
Calcium	41 mg
Iron	1.0 mg

- **Preheat oven to 350°F (180°C)**
- **13- by 9-inch (33 by 23 cm) glass baking dish, greased**

2	cloves garlic, minced	2
¼ cup	gluten-free cracker crumbs	60 mL
2 tbsp	chopped fresh parsley	30 mL
2 tbsp	olive oil (approx.)	30 mL
	Juice of ½ lemon	
3	pieces skinless sole fillet (each about 3½ oz/100 g)	3

1. In a small bowl, combine garlic, cracker crumbs, parsley, oil and lemon juice; stir until a paste forms, adding more oil if mixture is too dry.

2. Arrange sole in prepared baking dish. Spread paste over fish.

3. Cover dish with foil and bake in preheated oven for 20 to 30 minutes or until fish flakes easily when tested with a fork. Uncover and bake for 5 minutes or until crust is crispy.

Maple Ginger Salmon

Makes 4 servings

Nutrients per serving

Calories	319
Fat	12 g
Carbohydrate	14 g
Fiber	0 g
Protein	37 g
Calcium	47 mg
Iron	0.3 mg

- **Preheat oven to 350°F (180°C)**
- **Rimmed baking sheet, lined with foil**

4	skinless salmon fillets	4
¼ cup	pure maple syrup	60 mL
2 tbsp	cider vinegar or rice vinegar	30 mL
1 tsp	finely grated gingerroot	5 mL

1. Place salmon on prepared baking sheet.

2. In a small bowl, whisk together maple syrup, vinegar and ginger. Pour over fillets.

3. Bake in preheated oven for 10 to 15 minutes or until fish is opaque and flakes easily when tested with a fork.

Broiled Cilantro Ginger Salmon

Makes 6 servings

Broiling the fish on one side only keeps it moist, delicious and full of flavor.

Tips

This can also be cooked on a barbecue with two or more burners. Preheat one side to medium, place salmon on the other side and close the lid. This indirect cooking method is great for delicate proteins like fish. There will be enough heat to cook the salmon without burning it or drying it out.

Extra salmon is great served cold with a salad.

- **Rimmed baking sheet, greased**

3	cloves garlic, roughly chopped	3
2 tbsp	grated gingerroot	30 mL
½ tsp	salt	2 mL
½ cup	chopped fresh cilantro	125 mL
2 tbsp	olive oil	30 mL
½ tsp	freshly ground black pepper	2 mL
	Grated zest of 2 limes	
6	salmon fillets (about 2¼ lbs/1.125 kg total)	6

1. Using a mortar and pestle (or a food processor), crush garlic, ginger and salt to form a paste. Stir in cilantro, olive oil, pepper and lime zest.

2. Place salmon on a plate and coat top evenly with paste. Cover and refrigerate for at least 30 minutes or for up to 2 hours. Preheat broiler, with rack set 4 inches (10 cm) from the top.

3. Transfer salmon to prepared baking sheet and broil for 7 to 10 minutes or until salmon is opaque and flakes easily with a fork.

This recipe courtesy of Eileen Campbell.

Nutrients per serving

Calories	327
Fat	21 g
Carbohydrate	1 g
Fiber	0 g
Protein	30 g
Calcium	26 mg
Iron	0.6 mg

Smothered Salmon with Spinach

In this elegant recipe, salmon is smothered with seasonings, green onion and minced garlic, then poached in the oven on spinach leaves. Served with rice, this delicious dish makes a nourishing meal.

Tip

Refrigerate any leftovers in an airtight container for up to 2 days. Flake the fish and mix it with mayonnaise and sliced pickles or tartar sauce to make a sandwich filling, or serve chilled on top of a green salad.

- **Preheat oven to 325°F (160°C)**
- **13- by 9-inch (33 by 23 cm) baking dish**

12	large spinach leaves	12
2 lb	whole salmon	1 kg
1 tbsp	chopped fresh dill (or 1 tsp/5 mL dried dillweed)	15 mL
½ tsp	salt	2 mL
½ tsp	freshly ground black pepper	2 mL
1 cup	cold water	250 mL
1½ tsp	olive oil	7 mL
1	bunch green onions, sliced (about ⅔ cup/150 mL)	1
1	clove garlic, minced	1

1. Arrange spinach leaves on bottom of baking dish. Top with salmon; sprinkle with dill, salt and pepper. Pour water and oil over salmon. Top with green onions and garlic. Cover tightly with foil.

2. Bake in preheated oven for 25 to 30 minutes or until salmon flakes easily when tested with a fork, basting twice. Arrange salmon with spinach on serving platter with pan juices.

This recipe courtesy of chef Yvonne Levert and dietitian Nanette Porter-MacDonald.

Nutrients per serving

Calories	214
Fat	13 g
Carbohydrate	1 g
Fiber	0 g
Protein	23 g
Calcium	34 mg
Iron	0.7 mg

Mustard Maple Salmon with Watercress Quinoa

Makes 4 servings

With a nod to the Pacific Northwest, this super-quick mustard and maple glaze keeps the salmon fillets incredibly moist. A peppery bed of fresh watercress quinoa balances and brightens all.

Tip

If using ready-to-use broth for this recipe, make sure to purchase one that is gluten-free.

If wild salmon is unavailable, look for North American–farmed salmon (such as Coho, Sake or Silver), which is farmed in an environmentally friendly way.

Nutrients per serving

Calories	399
Fat	15 g
Carbohydrate	27 g
Fiber	3 g
Protein	38 g
Calcium	79 mg
Iron	3.0 mg

• **Preheat barbecue grill to medium-high**

¾ cup	quinoa, rinsed	175 mL
1½ cups	Chicken Stock (page 179), Vegetable Stock (page 178) or reduced-sodium ready-to-use chicken or vegetable broth	375 mL
1 tbsp	cider vinegar	15 mL
1 tbsp	pure maple syrup	15 mL
1 tbsp	extra virgin olive oil	15 mL
2 tsp	whole-grain Dijon mustard	10 mL
4	skinless wild salmon fillets (each about 5 oz/150 g)	4
	Nonstick cooking spray	
	Fine sea salt and freshly cracked black pepper	
3 cups	packed watercress sprigs	750 mL

1. In a medium saucepan, combine quinoa and stock. Bring to a boil over medium-high heat. Reduce heat to low, cover and simmer for 12 to 15 minutes or until liquid is absorbed. Remove from heat and let stand, covered, for 5 minutes. Fluff with a fork.

2. In a small bowl, whisk together vinegar, maple syrup, oil and mustard. Set aside.

3. Lightly spray both sides of fish with cooking spray, then sprinkle with salt and pepper. Grill on preheated barbecue, turning once, for 3 to 4 minutes per side or until fish is opaque and flakes easily when tested with a fork.

4. To the quinoa, add watercress, gently tossing to combine. Season to taste with salt and pepper. Serve salmon atop quinoa mixture, with maple mixture drizzled over fish.

Salmon Wraps

Makes 6 servings

These wraps are proof that the simplest recipes can yield the finest flavor.

Tips

Work quickly and carefully with the rice paper to be sure it does not tear or dry out.

Place cooled cooked parcels in a sealable plastic bag and freeze. Defrost in the microwave oven for a quick lunch.

- **Preheat oven to 375°F (190°C)**
- **Baking sheet, lightly greased**

6	8-inch (20 cm) rice paper rounds	6
6	sprigs fresh dill, stems removed	6
6	pieces skinless salmon fillet (about 1½ lbs/750 g total)	6
1	lemon, cut in half	1
Pinch	salt	Pinch

1. Fill a shallow dish with warm water. Lay out a clean, lint-free towel. Working with 1 round at a time, place rice paper in warm water for about 1 minute to soften. Carefully lift out of water and place on towel. Place 1 sprig fresh dill in the center of the round. Place 1 salmon fillet on top of dill. Sprinkle with a squeeze of lemon juice and a few grains of salt. Fold bottom half of rice paper up over salmon, fold in sides, then fold top down to enclose the salmon. Turn parcels over and place seam side down on prepared baking sheet. Repeat to make 6 parcels.

2. Bake in preheated oven for 10 to 12 minutes or until fish flakes easily when tested with a fork.

Variation

Use other fish, such as tilapia, haddock or cod, adjusting cooking times as needed.

This recipe courtesy of Judy Reynolds.

Nutrients per serving	
Calories	243
Fat	13 g
Carbohydrate	8 g
Fiber	0 g
Protein	24 g
Calcium	21 mg
Iron	0.5 mg

Lemon Dill Tilapia in Foil

Makes 4 servings

It doesn't get easier or more tasty than foil packets of tilapia with lemon, dill, parsley and olive oil!

Tip

Other mild, lean white fish, such as orange roughy, snapper, cod, tilefish or striped bass, may be used in place of the tilapia.

- **Preheat oven to 375°F (190°C)**
- **Four 12-inch (30 cm) squares foil**
- **Large rimmed baking sheet**

2	lemons, each cut into 6 slices	2
4	skinless farmed tilapia fillets (each about 6 oz/175 g)	4
½ tsp	fine sea salt, divided	2 mL
½ tsp	freshly cracked black pepper, divided	2 mL
½ cup	shredded carrot	125 mL
2 tbsp	chopped fresh dill	30 mL
2 tbsp	chopped fresh flat-leaf (Italian) parsley	30 mL
2 tsp	extra virgin olive oil	10 mL

1. Place foil squares on a work surface. Place 3 lemon slices in an overlapping line down the center of each square. Top each with a fish fillet and sprinkle with half the salt and half the pepper. Top with equal amounts of carrot, dill and parsley. Drizzle with oil and sprinkle with the remaining salt and pepper. Fold foil over fish and vegetables, crimping edges tightly to seal. Place packets on baking sheet.

2. Bake in preheated oven for 18 to 22 minutes or until fish is opaque and flakes easily when tested with a fork. Slide packets onto plates.

Nutrients per serving	
Calories	202
Fat	5 g
Carbohydrate	4 g
Fiber	2 g
Protein	35 g
Calcium	35 mg
Iron	1.2 mg

Broiled Herbed Trout Fillets

Butterflied trout fillets enhanced by a fresh herb dressing cook quickly under the broiler, delivering a light, satisfying entrée.

Tip

Other mild, lean white fish, such as orange roughy, snapper, cod, tilefish or striped bass, may be used in place of the trout.

- **Preheat broiler, with rack set 4 to 6 inches (10 to 15 cm) from the heat source**
- **Broiler pan, sprayed with nonstick cooking spray (preferably olive oil)**

1	clove garlic, minced	1
1 tbsp	minced fresh flat-leaf (Italian) parsley	15 mL
1 tbsp	minced fresh chives	15 mL
2 tsp	minced fresh oregano	10 mL
½ tsp	fine sea salt	2 mL
¼ tsp	freshly cracked black pepper	1 mL
1 tbsp	extra virgin olive oil	15 mL
1 tbsp	freshly squeezed lemon juice	15 mL
4	skin-on trout fillets (each about 6 oz/175 g)	4

1. In a medium bowl, whisk together garlic, parsley, chives, oregano, salt, pepper, oil and lemon juice.

2. Place fish, skin side down, on prepared pan. Generously brush with dressing. Broil for 4 to 6 minutes or until fish is opaque and flakes easily when tested with a fork.

Nutrients per serving

Calories	216
Fat	10 g
Carbohydrate	1 g
Fiber	0 g
Protein	30 g
Calcium	41 mg
Iron	0.7 mg

Indian-Spiced Lentils with Peppery Apricots

Makes 6 servings

Although the flavors are exotic, this qualifies as comfort food. Savory lentils seasoned with spices that are traditionally associated with the East are punctuated by sweet chewy apricots sprinkled with piquant cayenne.

Tip

If using ready-to-use broth for this recipe, make sure to purchase one that is gluten-free.

Make Ahead

Complete step 1. Cover and refrigerate for up to 2 days. When you're ready to cook, complete the recipe.

Nutrients per serving

Calories	298
Fat	4 g
Carbohydrate	58 g
Fiber	12 g
Protein	13 g
Calcium	98 mg
Iron	5.0 mg

• **Medium (minimum 4-quart) slow cooker**

1 tbsp	olive oil	15 mL
2	onions, finely chopped	2
4	stalks celery, diced	4
4	cloves garlic, minced	4
1 tbsp	minced gingerroot	15 mL
2 tsp	ground cumin	10 mL
2 tsp	ground coriander	10 mL
1 tsp	ground turmeric	5 mL
1	2-inch (5 cm) piece cinnamon stick	1
1½ cups	brown or green lentils, rinsed	375 mL
4 cups	Vegetable Stock (page 178) or reduced-sodium ready-to-use vegetable broth	1 L
1	sweet potato, peeled and diced	1
½ tsp	cayenne pepper	2 mL
1 cup	chopped dried apricots	250 mL
	Finely chopped fresh parsley	

1. In a skillet, heat oil over medium heat. Add onions and celery and cook, stirring, until softened, about 5 minutes. Add garlic, ginger, cumin, coriander, turmeric and cinnamon stick and cook, stirring, for 1 minute. Transfer to slow cooker stoneware. Stir in lentils and stock.

2. Add sweet potato and stir well. Cover and cook on Low for 6 to 8 hours or on High for 3 to 4 hours, until lentils are tender.

3. In a small bowl, sprinkle cayenne evenly over apricots. Add to stoneware and stir well. Cover and cook on High for 15 minutes to meld flavors. Discard cinnamon stick. Garnish with parsley.

Vegetable Curry with Lentils and Spinach

Serve this delicious curry for dinner with warm Indian bread such as naan. It's a meal in itself.

Tips

If using ready-to-use broth for this recipe, make sure to purchase one that is gluten-free.

If using fresh spinach, be sure to remove the stems, and if it has not been prewashed, rinse it thoroughly in a basin of lukewarm water.

Nutrients per serving

Calories	252
Fat	3 g
Carbohydrate	50 g
Fiber	9 g
Protein	10 g
Calcium	118 mg
Iron	4.5 mg

• **Large (minimum 5 quart) slow cooker**

2 tsp	cumin seeds	10 mL
1 tsp	coriander seeds	5 mL
1 tbsp	olive oil or extra virgin coconut oil	15 mL
2	onions, finely chopped	2
4	carrots, peeled and thinly sliced (about 1 lb/500 g)	4
4	parsnips, peeled, tough core removed and thinly sliced (about 1 lb/500 g)	4
4	cloves garlic, minced	4
1 tbsp	minced gingerroot	15 mL
2 tsp	ground turmeric	10 mL
1	2-inch (5 cm) cinnamon stick	1
½ tsp	cracked black peppercorns	2 mL
2 cups	Vegetable Stock (page 178) or reduced-sodium ready-to-use vegetable broth	500 mL
	Salt (optional)	
2	sweet potatoes, peeled and thinly sliced (about 1 lb/500 g)	2
1 cup	brown or green lentils, picked over and rinsed	250 mL
1	long red chile pepper, finely chopped (or ½ tsp/2 mL cayenne pepper, dissolved in 1 tbsp/15 mL lemon juice)	1
1 lb	fresh spinach, stems removed (or one 10-oz/300 g package spinach leaves, thawed and drained if frozen, coarsely chopped)	500 g
1 cup	coconut milk (optional)	250 mL

Tip

The coconut milk adds
a pleasant nutty flavor
and creaminess to
the curry, but it is high
in saturated fat. So if
you're concerned about
your intake of saturated
fat, leave it out. The
curry is very tasty on
its own.

Make Ahead

This dish can be
partially prepared
before it is cooked.
Complete steps 1 and
2. Cover and refrigerate
overnight or for up to
2 days. When you're
ready to cook, continue
with step 3.

1. In a dry skillet over medium heat, toast cumin and coriander seeds until fragrant and cumin seeds just begin to brown, about 3 minutes. Immediately transfer to a mortar or a spice grinder and grind. Set aside.

2. In same skillet, heat oil over medium heat for 30 seconds. Add onions, carrots and parsnips and cook, stirring, until vegetables are tender, about 6 minutes. Add garlic, gingerroot, turmeric, cinnamon stick, peppercorns and reserved cumin and coriander and cook, stirring, for 1 minute. Add stock and bring to a boil. Season to taste with salt (if using) and transfer to slow cooker stoneware. Add sweet potatoes and lentils and stir well.

3. Cover and cook on Low for 8 hours or on High for 4 hours, until lentils are tender. Add chile pepper and stir well. Add spinach, in batches, stirring after each batch until all the leaves are submerged in the liquid, then coconut milk, if using. Cover and cook on High for 20 minutes, until spinach is wilted and flavors have blended. Discard cinnamon stick.

Red Lentil Curry with Coconut and Cilantro

Easy to make, these red lentils have a luxurious coconut finish. To reduce your caloric intake, make this recipe with light coconut milk. Choose enriched coconut milk to increase your intake of calcium and vitamin D.

Tips

Try using extra virgin olive oil instead of vegetable oil.

Traditionally, Indian lentil dishes are served almost soupy. You can adjust the texture to your taste by adding more water or simmering longer to thicken in step 2.

Nutrients per serving		
Calories	288	
Fat	19 g	
Carbohydrate	22 g	
Fiber	5 g	
Protein	10 g	
Calcium	35 mg	
Iron	4.1 mg	

2 tbsp	vegetable oil	30 mL
1	small onion, finely chopped	1
2	cloves garlic, minced	2
1 tbsp	minced gingerroot	15 mL
	Salt	
1 tsp	ground coriander	5 mL
1 tsp	ground cumin	5 mL
¼ tsp	ground turmeric	1 mL
1 cup	dried red lentils (masoor dal), rinsed	250 mL
1	can (14 oz/400 mL) coconut milk	1
1 cup	water	250 mL
¼ cup	torn fresh cilantro leaves	60 mL
	Garam masala	

1. In a saucepan, heat oil over medium heat. Add onion and cook, stirring, until softened and starting to brown, about 5 minutes. Add garlic, ginger, 1 tsp (5 mL) salt, coriander, cumin and turmeric; cook, stirring, until softened and fragrant, about 2 minutes.

2. Stir in lentils until coated with spices. Stir in coconut milk and water; bring to a boil, scraping up bits stuck to pan and stirring to prevent lumps. Reduce heat to low, partially cover and simmer, stirring often, until lentils are very soft and mixture is thick, about 15 minutes.

3. Remove from heat, cover and let stand for 5 minutes. Season to taste with salt. Stir in all but a few leaves of cilantro. Serve sprinkled with remaining cilantro and garam masala.

Variation

To add some heat to this dish, add 1 or 2 hot red or green chile peppers, minced, with the garlic.

Sweet Potato and Spinach Curry with Quinoa

If you've never had sweet potatoes in a curry dish before, you'll be surprised by how well they take to bold spices. Coconut milk and quinoa act as dual complements, stealthily rounding out the interplay of sweet and umami that will have you savoring every last bite.

Tips

If using ready-to-use broth for this recipe, make sure to purchase one that is gluten-free.

Try using extra virgin olive oil instead of vegetable oil.

Nutrients per serving	
Calories	411
Fat	17 g
Carbohydrate	59 g
Fiber	10 g
Protein	10 g
Calcium	106 mg
Iron	6.4 mg

1 cup	quinoa, rinsed	250 mL
3½ cups	Vegetable Stock (page 178) or reduced-sodium ready-to-use vegetable broth, divided	875 mL
2 tsp	vegetable oil	10 mL
1	large onion, thinly sliced	1
2 tbsp	mild curry powder	30 mL
⅛ tsp	cayenne pepper	0.5 mL
2 lbs	sweet potatoes, peeled and cut into 1-inch (2.5 cm) chunks	1 kg
1	can (14 oz/400 mL) light coconut milk	1
8 cups	packed baby spinach (about 6 oz/175 g)	2 L
1 tbsp	freshly squeezed lime juice	15 mL
	Fine sea salt and ground black pepper	

1. In a medium saucepan, combine quinoa and 2 cups (500 mL) of the stock. Bring to a boil over medium-high heat. Reduce heat to low, cover and simmer for 12 to 15 minutes or until liquid is absorbed. Remove from heat and let stand, covered, for 5 minutes. Fluff with a fork.

2. Meanwhile, in a large saucepan, heat oil over medium-high heat. Add onion and cook, stirring, for 6 to 8 minutes or until softened. Add curry powder and cayenne; cook, stirring, for 30 seconds.

3. Stir in sweet potatoes and the remaining stock; bring to a boil. Reduce heat and boil for 12 minutes. Add coconut milk, reduce heat and simmer, stirring occasionally, for 3 to 7 minutes or until sweet potatoes are tender. Stir in spinach and lime juice; simmer for 1 to 2 minutes or until spinach is wilted. Season to taste with salt and pepper. Serve over quinoa.

Quinoa Vegetable Stir-Fry

Quinoa is a delicious Peruvian nut-like grain. Combined with a legume, such as lima beans, it is an great alternative to meat. It is high in fiber and an excellent source of iron.

1 cup	quinoa, rinsed	250 mL
1	package (12 oz/350 g) frozen lima beans	1
1 cup	thinly sliced carrots	250 mL
1 tbsp	vegetable oil	15 mL
	Salt and freshly ground black pepper	

1. Rinse quinoa under cold running water until water is clear. In a medium saucepan, bring quinoa and 1 cup (250 mL) water to a boil. Reduce heat. Cover and cook for 15 minutes or until tender. Drain and transfer to bowl.

2. In same saucepan, add a small amount of water to lima beans and carrots. Bring to a boil. Reduce heat and cook for 5 minutes or until vegetables are tender. Drain.

3. In a wok or frying pan, heat oil. Add quinoa, cooked vegetables and salt and pepper. Stir-fry until heated.

Nutrients per serving

Calories	316
Fat	6 g
Carbohydrate	52 g
Fiber	9 g
Protein	13 g
Calcium	73 mg
Iron	3.6 mg

Chicken, Turkey and Lamb

Roast Chicken with Leeks

This easy-to-prepare meal is a delicious and nutrient-rich variation on a classic favorite.

Tip

You can use Chicken Stock (page 179), gluten-free ready-to-use chicken broth or wine instead of water, if desired.

- **Preheat oven to 325°F (160°C)**
- **Roasting pan**

1	roasting chicken (about 3 lbs/1.5 kg)	1
1	lemon, quartered	1
6	cloves garlic, sliced	6
2	large leeks, trimmed and washed	2
	Salt and freshly ground black pepper	

1. Rinse and wipe chicken with paper towel. Place breast side down in roasting pan. Stuff cavity with lemon and garlic.

2. Slice leeks in half lengthwise. Place cut side down in roasting pan alongside chicken. Sprinkle with salt and pepper. Pour in $\frac{3}{4}$ cup (175 mL) water (see tip, at left). Cover tightly.

3. Roast in preheated oven for 40 minutes. Remove from oven and transfer leeks to a dish and keep warm. Return chicken to oven. Continue roasting, uncovered, for about $1\frac{1}{2}$ hours or until meat thermometer registers 180°F (82°C). Remove chicken from oven. Let stand for 5 minutes before carving. Serve with leeks and any pan juices.

Nutrients per serving

Calories	195
Fat	8 g
Carbohydrate	2 g
Fiber	0 g
Protein	28 g
Calcium	9 mg
Iron	0.3 mg

Lemon-Thyme Roast Chicken

A roast chicken that is crispy on the outside and juicy on the inside is hard to beat.

Tip

Using a V-shaped rack is an excellent and healthy way to roast chicken. The open cavity of the chicken is placed over the rack, allowing the chicken to roast upright. If you don't have a V-shaped rack, you can just place the chicken in the roasting pan. However, the overall result is better with the rack — the chicken skin crisps all around, and any excess fat drips off into the pan.

- **Roasting pan with V-shaped rack**

1	roasting chicken (5 to 6 lbs/2.5 to 3 kg)	1
4	cloves garlic, minced	4
¼ cup	olive oil	60 mL
2 tbsp	chopped fresh thyme	30 mL
1 tsp	freshly ground black pepper	5 mL
	Grated zest and juice of 1 lemon	
	Salt	

1. Prepare chicken by trimming excess fat from body or cavity. Rinse inside and out under cold running water and pat dry.

2. In a bowl large enough to hold the chicken, whisk together garlic, olive oil, thyme, pepper, lemon zest, lemon juice and salt to taste. Place chicken in bowl and turn to coat completely, inside and out. Cover and refrigerate for at least 1 hour or overnight. Preheat oven to 450°F (230°C) and remove top rack.

3. Place chicken on rack in roasting pan and baste with marinade. Roast for 15 to 20 minutes. Reduce heat to 375°F (190°C) and roast for 1½ to 2 hours (depending on the size of the chicken) or until skin is dark golden and crispy, drumsticks wiggle when touched, and a meat thermometer inserted into the thickest part of a thigh registers 185°F (85°C). Remove from oven and let rest, tented with foil, for 10 to 15 minutes before carving. (This allows the juices to redistribute and provides a much moister chicken.)

Variations

Try other seasoning combinations for this roast chicken. Make it international by using tandoori paste or a mixture of hoisin and chili sauces.

For a one-dish meal, add cubed root vegetables, such as sweet potatoes, carrots, potatoes and turnips, around the chicken for the last hour of cooking. For the last 10 minutes of cooking, add apple or pear slices.

This recipe courtesy of Eileen Campbell.

Nutrients per serving	
Calories	231
Fat	15 g
Carbohydrate	1 g
Fiber	0 g
Protein	24 g
Calcium	14 mg
Iron	1.0 mg

Baked Chicken with Lemon Herb Sauce

Makes 8 servings

Nutrients per serving

Calories	104
Fat	2 g
Carbohydrate	2 g
Fiber	0 g
Protein	19 g
Calcium	11 mg
Iron	1.1 mg

¼ cup	freshly squeezed lemon juice	60 mL
¼ cup	chopped fresh oregano	60 mL
¼ cup	chopped fresh chives	60 mL
	Salt and freshly ground black pepper	
8	chicken pieces, such as breasts or drumsticks	8

1. Stir together lemon juice, oregano, chives and salt and pepper. Pour into a serving dish large enough to hold all chicken pieces.

2. Rinse and wipe chicken with paper towel. Grill at medium-high heat or roast until meat is no longer pink inside, about 20 minutes.

3. When chicken is cooked, transfer to bowl with lemon mixture. Turn to coat and serve.

Mustard-Lime Chicken

Makes 4 servings

Nutrients per serving

Calories	183
Fat	2 g
Carbohydrate	21 g
Fiber	0 g
Protein	19 g
Calcium	0 mg
Iron	1.1 mg

• **Preheat barbecue to medium-high**

2	limes, divided	2
¼ cup	Dijon mustard	60 mL
¼ cup	liquid honey	60 mL
4	boneless skinless chicken breasts	4

1. Cut one lime into slices. Set aside. Grate zest and squeeze out juice from remaining lime. Place lime zest and juice in a small bowl. Whisk in mustard and honey.

2. Rinse and wipe chicken with paper towel. Cook chicken on preheated grill for 7 minutes per side, brushing often with mustard mixture. Grill until meat is no longer pink inside.

3. Serve with any remaining sauce and lime slices.

Apple Harvest Chicken

Everyone will enjoy this fast and tasty chicken recipe. Serve with green beans and mashed potatoes for a simple weeknight dinner.

	Nonstick cooking spray	
4	boneless skinless chicken breasts	4
½ tsp	dried thyme	2 mL
	Salt and freshly ground black pepper	
2	medium apples, peeled and thickly sliced	2
¼ cup	apple cider or apple juice	60 mL

1. Rinse and wipe chicken with paper towel. Sprinkle with thyme, salt and pepper.

2. In a large nonstick skillet lightly sprayed with cooking spray, sauté chicken on medium-high for 5 minutes on each side or until browned.

3. Add apples and cider. Cover, reduce heat to medium-low and cook gently for 10 minutes or until meat is no longer pink inside.

Nutrients per serving

Calories	155
Fat	2 g
Carbohydrate	16 g
Fiber	2 g
Protein	19 g
Calcium	8 mg
Iron	1.4 mg

Grilled Garlic-Ginger Chicken Breasts

Tips

Broiler Method: After removing chicken from marinade, place in a lightly greased 9-inch (23 cm) square baking pan and pour in marinade. Broil, turning once, for 5 to 6 minutes per side or until chicken is no longer pink inside and has reached an internal temperature of 170°F (77°C).

Extra cooked chicken is always useful to add a quick protein boost to salads, stir-fries and soups.

2 tbsp	freshly squeezed lemon juice	30 mL
2 tsp	minced garlic	10 mL
2 tsp	minced gingerroot	10 mL
2 tsp	olive oil	10 mL
1 tsp	ground cumin	5 mL
4	boneless skinless chicken breasts (1 lb/500 g total)	4
	Freshly ground black pepper	

1. In a shallow dish, whisk together lemon juice, garlic, ginger, olive oil and cumin. Add chicken and turn to coat. Let stand at room temperature for 10 minutes, or cover and refrigerate for up to 4 hours. Preheat barbecue to medium.

2. Remove chicken from marinade and discard marinade. Place chicken on barbecue and cook, turning once, for 3 to 5 minutes per side or until chicken is no longer pink inside and has reached an internal temperature of 170°F (77°C). Season to taste with pepper.

This recipe courtesy of Judy Jenkins.

Nutrients per serving

Calories	145
Fat	3 g
Carbohydrate	1 g
Fiber	0 g
Protein	26 g
Calcium	11 mg
Iron	0.8 mg

Spring Vegetable Chicken Quinoa

Makes 6 servings

Quinoa adds a stick-to-the-ribs earthiness to this chicken dish, while peas, asparagus and lemon render it just right for spring.

Tip

An equal amount of fresh mint or cilantro leaves may be used in place of the parsley.

1 tbsp	extra virgin olive oil	15 mL
6	green onions, thinly sliced crosswise, white and green parts separated	6
1 cup	quinoa, rinsed	250 mL
2 tsp	finely grated lemon zest	10 mL
¾ tsp	fine sea salt	3 mL
½ tsp	freshly cracked black pepper	2 mL
2 cups	water	500 mL
1 lb	asparagus, trimmed and cut into ½-inch (1 cm) pieces	500 g
2 cups	diced cooked chicken breast	500 mL
⅔ cup	frozen petite peas, thawed	150 mL
1 tbsp	freshly squeezed lemon juice	15 mL
¼ cup	packed fresh flat-leaf (Italian) parsley leaves, chopped	60 mL

1. In a medium saucepan, heat oil over medium-high heat. Add white parts of green onions and cook, stirring, for 2 to 3 minutes or until softened.

2. Stir in quinoa, lemon zest, salt, pepper and water. Bring to a boil. Reduce heat to low, cover and simmer for 11 minutes. Stir in asparagus, cover and simmer for 4 to 5 minutes or until liquid is absorbed and quinoa and asparagus are tender.

3. Remove from heat and stir in chicken, peas and lemon juice. Cover and let stand for 2 minutes to warm through. Stir in parsley and green parts of green onions.

Nutrients per serving	
Calories	253
Fat	6 g
Carbohydrate	27 g
Fiber	5 g
Protein	24 g
Calcium	56 mg
Iron	3.3 mg

Grilled Chicken Kabobs

Put the chicken in the fridge to marinate first thing in the morning. Then, at suppertime, all you have to do is thread the chicken onto skewers and grill the kabobs. Serve with tzatziki on the side.

• **Four 8- or 9-inch (20 or 23 cm) metal or wooden skewers**

2 to 3	cloves garlic, minced	2 to 3
1½ tbsp	olive oil	22 mL
1 tsp	dried parsley	5 mL
½ tsp	dried oregano	2 mL
1 lb	boneless skinless chicken breasts, cut into 1½-inch (4 cm) cubes	500 g
	Salt and freshly ground black pepper	

1. In a large sealable plastic bag, combine garlic to taste, oil, parsley and oregano. Add chicken, seal and toss to coat. Refrigerate for at least 6 hours or overnight.

2. Preheat barbecue grill to medium. If using wooden skewers, soak them in water for 10 minutes.

3. Remove chicken from marinade, discarding marinade. Thread chicken onto skewers, leaving space between pieces. Grill chicken, turning often, for 7 to 10 minutes per side or until chicken is no longer pink inside. Season to taste with salt and pepper.

Nutrients per serving

Calories	180
Fat	7 g
Carbohydrate	1 g
Fiber	0 g
Protein	26 g
Calcium	19 mg
Iron	1.0 mg

Herb Roast Turkey Roll

Turkey adapts readily to added flavorings, especially to herbs, spices and garlic. The finished roast carves into neat slices to enjoy hot or cold.

• **Preheat oven to 325°F (160°C)**

1	turkey roll (about 4 lbs/2 kg)	1
10	large cloves garlic, minced	10
3 tbsp	chopped fresh rosemary (or 1 tbsp/15 mL dried)	45 mL
1 tsp	salt	5 mL
¼ tsp	freshly ground black pepper	1 mL
2 tbsp	olive oil	30 mL

1. Place turkey roll on a cutting board and unroll as flat as possible.

2. In a small bowl, combine garlic, rosemary, salt, pepper and oil. Spread half of mixture over inside of turkey. Reroll and tie firmly with string. Spread remaining mixture over outside of roll.

3. Roast on a rack in preheated oven for $1\frac{1}{2}$ hours or until a meat thermometer registers 180°F (82°C). Remove from oven and let stand for 10 minutes before carving.

**Nutrients
per serving**

Calories	296
Fat	12 g
Carbohydrate	10 g
Fiber	0 g
Protein	35 g
Calcium	66 mg
Iron	2.6 mg

BBQ Butterflied Leg of Lamb

This simple Greek-style marinade is the perfect companion to grilled lamb, which is best served medium-rare.

Tips

Ask your butcher to prepare a butterflied leg of lamb for you. You may need to order it a day or two in advance.

A serving size of meat should be about 2 to 3 oz (60 to 90 g), about the size of the palm of your hand.

1	2-lb (1 kg) butterflied leg of lamb, trimmed	1
1 tsp	minced garlic	5 mL
2 tbsp	lemon juice	30 mL
2 tbsp	chopped fresh oregano (or 2 tsp/10 mL dried)	30 mL
2 tbsp	chopped fresh mint (or 2 tsp/10 mL dried)	30 mL
1 tbsp	olive oil	15 mL
	Freshly ground black pepper	

1. Place lamb in a large shallow dish, fat side down. Spread with garlic. Sprinkle with lemon juice, oregano, mint and olive oil. Season to taste with pepper.

2. Cover and marinate in refrigerator, turning once or twice, for 2 hours or overnight. Remove from refrigerator 30 minutes before grilling.

3. Preheat barbecue or broiler. For medium-rare, barbecue on greased grill for 10 to 12 minutes per side, depending on thickness of lamb or, if using a meat thermometer, until the internal temperature of lamb registers 140° to 150°F (60° to 65°C).

This recipe courtesy of dietitian Bev Callaghan.

Nutrients per serving

Calories	177
Fat	7 g
Carbohydrate	1 g
Fiber	0 g
Protein	26 g
Calcium	18 mg
Iron	2.8 mg

Middle Eastern Lamb, Greens and Quinoa

Ground lamb and Middle Eastern spices add deep flavor to a simple dish of chickpeas and chard; quinoa absorbs the flavorful juices.

Tips

If using ready-to-use broth for this recipe, make sure to purchase one that is gluten-free.

Try drizzling the finished dish with coconut milk instead of yogurt.

1	large bunch red Swiss chard	1
8 oz	lean or extra-lean ground lamb	250 g
4	cloves garlic, minced	4
2 tbsp	minced gingerroot	30 mL
1½ tsp	ground cumin	7 mL
1 tsp	ground coriander	5 mL
¼ tsp	cayenne pepper	1 mL
½ cup	Chicken Stock (page 179), Vegetable Stock (page 178) or reduced-sodium ready-to-use chicken or vegetable broth	125 mL
1	can (14 to 19 oz/398 to 540 mL) chickpeas, drained and rinsed	1
2 tsp	finely grated lemon zest	10 mL
2 tbsp	freshly squeezed lemon juice	30 mL
	Fine sea salt and freshly cracked black pepper	
3 cups	hot cooked quinoa	750 mL
¾ cup	plain yogurt	175 mL

1. Trim off tough stems from Swiss chard and discard. Trim tender stems and ribs from leaves and finely chop stems and ribs. Thinly slice leaves crosswise (to measure about 5 cups/1.25 L).

2. In a large, deep skillet, cook lamb, garlic, ginger, cumin, coriander and cayenne over medium-high heat, breaking lamb up with a spoon, for 5 to 6 minutes or until lamb is no longer pink.

3. Stir in Swiss chard and stock; cook, stirring, for 3 to 4 minutes or until Swiss chard is just wilted. Stir in chickpeas, lemon zest and lemon juice; cook, tossing, for 2 to 3 minutes to warm through and blend the flavors. Season to taste with salt and black pepper.

4. Divide quinoa among four dinner plates and top with lamb mixture. Drizzle with yogurt.

Nutrients per serving

Calories	438
Fat	14 g
Carbohydrate	52 g
Fiber	9 g
Protein	27 g
Calcium	167 mg
Iron	6.0 mg

Lamb Souvlaki

In this Greek favorite, chunks of lamb are marinated in a lemon juice, oil and herb mixture before being skewered and grilled. Vegetable chunks, such as green pepper or onion, can be added.

Tip

If you are basting with the lemon marinade in which the raw meat has been marinating, bring it to a boil for 5 minutes to kill any harmful bacteria left from marinating raw meat.

● **Wooden skewers, soaked in cold water for 10 minutes**

1 lb	lean boneless lamb	500 g
¼ cup	freshly squeezed lemon juice	60 mL
¼ cup	olive oil	60 mL
2 to 4	cloves garlic, minced	2 to 4
	Salt and freshly ground black pepper	

1. Trim lamb and discard fat. Cut into 1-inch (2.5 cm) chunks. Set aside.

2. In a bowl, whisk together lemon juice, oil, garlic, salt and pepper. Add meat and stir to coat. Marinate for up to 24 hours in the refrigerator or at room temperature for 30 minutes.

3. Remove meat from marinade. Reserve marinade for basting (see tip, at left).

4. Thread meat on four skewers. Broil under preheated broiler 6 inches (15 cm) from heat. Turn and baste halfway through with cooked marinade. Or grill on preheated broiler over medium-high heat for 5 minutes per side for rare and 7 minutes per side for medium.

Nutrients per serving

Calories	355
Fat	25 g
Carbohydrate	2 g
Fiber	0 g
Protein	30 g
Calcium	23 mg
Iron	2.8 mg

Side Dishes

Green Beans with Cashews

The simple addition of cashews and red onions transforms ordinary green beans into a delightful companion to any main course. Cashews are rich in heart-protective monounsaturated fats and the bone-strengthening mineral magnesium.

1 lb	green beans, trimmed	500 g
2 tbsp	olive oil	30 mL
½ cup	slivered red onion	125 mL
⅓ cup	raw cashews	75 mL
¼ tsp	salt	1 mL
¼ tsp	freshly ground black pepper	1 mL
	Few sprigs fresh parsley, chopped	

1. Blanch green beans in a pot of boiling water for 5 minutes. Drain and immediately refresh in a bowl of ice-cold water. Drain and set aside.

2. In a large skillet, heat olive oil over medium-high heat for 30 seconds. Add onions, cashews, salt and pepper and stir-fry for 2 to 3 minutes, until the onions are softened. Add cooked green beans, increase heat to high, and stir-fry actively for 2 to 3 minutes, until the beans feel hot to the touch. (Take care that you don't burn any cashews in the process.) Transfer to a serving plate and garnish with chopped parsley. Serve immediately.

Nutrients per serving

Calories	519
Fat	13 g
Carbohydrate	76 g
Fiber	3 g
Protein	29 g
Calcium	9 mg
Iron	0.8 mg

Roasted Beets with Carrots

Makes 4 servings

Substantial vegetables with a lot of flavor and fiber, such as beets and carrots, are the best candidates for roasting. Although the roasting of the two vegetables takes a little over an hour, the end results are simply superb. In fact, the beets can be completed up to 2 days ahead, chilled and finished just before serving.

- **Preheat oven to 425°F (220°C)**
- **Baking dish, greased**

3	medium beets, trimmed	3
3	medium carrots, peeled and cut diagonally into ¾-inch (2 cm) slices	3
2 tbsp	olive oil	30 mL
	Salt and freshly ground black pepper	

1. Wrap beets tightly with foil into one large package. Roast for $1\frac{1}{4}$ hours or until beets are tender.

2. Meanwhile, toss carrots with oil, salt and pepper. Place in a shallow baking dish and roast in preheated oven for 20 minutes or until almost tender. Remove vegetables from oven.

3. When beets are cool enough to handle, open foil and remove skin. Cut each into 8 wedges.

4. Add beets to carrots and toss to combine. Roast for 15 minutes more or until beets are hot and carrots are very tender.

Variation

Roasted Cauliflower: Replace beets and carrots with 1 large cauliflower, broken into small florets. Combine oil, 1 tsp (5 mL) chopped fresh rosemary, salt and pepper. Toss with cauliflower to coat. Place in a single layer on a greased baking dish. Bake in a 400°F (200°C) preheated oven for 25 minutes or until cooked through and lightly browned.

Nutrients per serving

Calories	105
Fat	7 g
Carbohydrate	10 g
Fiber	3 g
Protein	1 g
Calcium	25 mg
Iron	0.7 mg

Quick Sautéed Kale

Kale is a bona fide superfood, high in antioxidants, such as vitamin A and C, as well as important nutrients such as vitamin B_6, calcium and magnesium. Enjoy!

Tip

Try using cider vinegar instead of the red wine vinegar.

• **Steamer basket**

1 lb	kale, tough stems and ribs removed, leaves cut into ¼-inch (0.5 cm) wide strips (about 8 cups/2 L)	500 g
1 tbsp	extra virgin olive oil	15 mL
1 cup	thinly sliced red onion	250 mL
2	cloves garlic, minced	2
Pinch	hot pepper flakes	Pinch
¼ tsp	fine sea salt	1 mL
1 tbsp	red wine vinegar	15 mL

1. Place kale in steamer basket set over a large pot of boiling water. Cover and steam for 8 to 10 minutes or until tender.

2. In a large skillet, heat oil over medium-high heat. Add red onion and cook, stirring, for 6 to 8 minutes or until golden. Add garlic and hot pepper flakes; cook, stirring, for 1 minute. Add kale, reduce heat to medium and cook, stirring occasionally, for 1 to 2 minutes or until heated through. Remove from heat and stir in salt and vinegar.

Nutrients per serving

Calories	86
Fat	3 g
Carbohydrate	14 g
Fiber	3 g
Protein	4 g
Calcium	245 mg
Iron	3.5 mg

Spinach with Almonds

Did you know that cooked spinach has more iron than raw spinach? And you can up the iron even more by topping it off with almonds.

1	package (10 oz/300 g) fresh spinach, trimmed	1
2 tbsp	olive oil	30 mL
½ cup	slivered almonds	125 mL
	Salt and freshly ground black pepper	

1. Rinse spinach under cold running water. In a large saucepan, over medium-high heat, cook spinach in the water clinging to the leaves, stirring, for 3 to 5 minutes or until wilted. Drain and transfer to a serving platter.

2. Drizzle oil over spinach and sprinkle with almonds. Season to taste with salt and pepper.

Nutrients per serving

Calories	140
Fat	12 g
Carbohydrate	5 g
Fiber	3 g
Protein	5 g
Calcium	106 mg
Iron	2.0 mg

Wilted Spinach with Garlic

This easy-to-prepare vegetable side dish is full of nutrients and flavor.

Tips

Try using cider vinegar instead of the sherry or red wine vinegar.

Spinach is iron-rich, and garlic lowers cholesterol and blood pressure.

2 tsp	extra virgin olive oil	10 mL
3	cloves garlic, thinly sliced lengthwise	3
2	packages (each 10 oz/300 g) baby spinach	2
1 tbsp	water	15 mL
1/8 tsp	fine sea salt	0.5 mL
1/8 tsp	freshly ground black pepper	0.5 mL
1/2 tsp	sherry vinegar or red wine vinegar	2 mL

1. In a large pot, heat oil over medium-high heat. Add garlic, spinach and water; cook, tossing with tongs, for about 2 minutes or until spinach is wilted but still bright green. Add salt, pepper and vinegar, gently tossing to combine.

Nutrients per serving

Calories	57
Fat	2 g
Carbohydrate	11 g
Fiber	5 g
Protein	3 g
Calcium	73 mg
Iron	3.2 mg

Sautéed Spinach with Pine Nuts

This is an easy way to add flavor to spinach. You can substitute Swiss chard, kale, rapini or mustard greens for the spinach and increase the cooking time accordingly. If you don't have pine nuts, try chopped pecans or walnuts.

Tip

Stir-frying vegetables is a great way to preserve nutrients. When boiled, vegetables can lose up to 45% of their vitamin C, compared with a loss of only 5% when stir-fried.

2 tsp	olive oil	10 mL
¼ cup	pine nuts	60 mL
1	package (10 oz/300 g) fresh spinach, trimmed	1
1 tsp	minced garlic	5 mL
1 tsp	freshly squeezed lemon juice	5 mL
⅛ tsp	ground nutmeg	0.5 mL
	Freshly ground black pepper	

1. In a large nonstick skillet, heat 1 tsp (5 mL) of the oil over medium heat. Add pine nuts and cook, stirring constantly, for 2 to 3 minutes or until golden. Remove pine nuts from pan and set aside.

2. Add remaining oil to pan. Add spinach in several bunches (it will cook down quickly), stirring constantly. Add garlic and cook, stirring, for 1 to 2 minutes, until fragrant. Stir in lemon juice and nutmeg. Season to taste with pepper. Add reserved pine nuts. Cook until heated through.

This recipe courtesy of dietitian Bev Callaghan.

Nutrients per serving

Calories	109
Fat	8 g
Carbohydrate	9 g
Fiber	4 g
Protein	3 g
Calcium	56 mg
Iron	2.9 mg

Sautéed Swiss Chard

Makes 8 servings

Earthy, grassy Swiss chard makes a gorgeous, incredibly tasty side dish. It needs little adornment beyond a bit of olive oil and garlic.

3 lbs	Swiss chard (about 2 large bunches)	1.5 kg
1 tbsp	extra virgin olive oil	15 mL
2	onions, halved, then thinly sliced	2
3	cloves garlic, minced	3
¼ tsp	fine sea salt	1 mL
¼ tsp	freshly ground black pepper	1 mL

1. Trim stems and center ribs from Swiss chard, then cut stems and ribs crosswise into 1-inch (2.5 cm) pieces. Stack chard leaves, roll them up crosswise into a tight cylinder and cut the cylinder crosswise into 1-inch (2.5 cm) thick slices.

2. In a large, heavy pot, heat oil over medium heat. Add onions and cook, stirring, for 8 to 9 minutes or until golden. Stir in chard stems and ribs, garlic, salt and pepper. Cover and cook, stirring occasionally, for 8 to 10 minutes or until stems are tender.

3. Add half the chard leaves and cook, stirring, for 1 minute or until slightly wilted. Add the remaining leaves, cover and cook, stirring occasionally, for 4 to 6 minutes or until leaves are tender. Using a slotted spoon, transfer Swiss chard mixture to plates or a serving bowl.

Nutrients per serving

Calories	52
Fat	1 g
Carbohydrate	10 g
Fiber	4 g
Protein	4 g
Calcium	107 mg
Iron	3.9 mg

Skillet-Style Onion and Sweet Potatoes

Eye appeal and great taste make this vegetable dish a pleasing addition to the dinner plate. Vitamin C and beta carotene make it very nutritious. And it can be prepared in very short order!

Tip

If using ready-to-use broth for this recipe, make sure to purchase one that is gluten-free.

1 tbsp	olive oil	15 mL
1	large onion, sliced	1
2	large sweet potatoes, peeled and thinly sliced	2
2/3 cup	Vegetable Stock (page 178) or reduced-sodium ready-to-use vegetable broth	150 mL
	Salt and freshly ground black pepper	

1. In a nonstick skillet, heat oil over medium heat. Cook onion, stirring frequently, for 5 minutes or until soft.
2. Add potatoes and stock. Cover and bring to a boil. Reduce heat to medium-low and cook slowly, stirring frequently, for 15 minutes or until potatoes are tender. Season lightly with salt and pepper.

Nutrients per serving

Calories	129
Fat	4 g
Carbohydrate	23 g
Fiber	4 g
Protein	2 g
Calcium	47 mg
Iron	0.8 mg

Roasted Butternut Squash

The wonderful aroma of baking squash is so appealing. Try roasting it with some olive oil. The aromas are even better. So is the taste!

Tip

Tossing ingredients of an oily nature in a clean plastic bag makes for short and easy cleanup. If your milk comes in heavy individual bags, cut one end of an emptied bag, wash and reuse for this purpose.

- **Preheat oven to 400°F (200°C)**
- **Baking pan, lined with foil**

1	medium butternut squash, peeled	1
1 to 2 tsp	minced fresh gingerroot	5 to 10 mL
1	large clove garlic, minced	1
1 tbsp	olive oil	15 mL
	Salt and freshly ground black pepper	

1. Cut squash into bite-size cubes.

2. In a large bowl or plastic bag (see tip, at left), toss squash, gingerroot, garlic, oil, salt and pepper.

3. Arrange on prepared baking pan in a single layer. Bake in preheated oven, stirring occasionally, for 40 minutes or until tender and starting to brown.

Nutrients per serving

Calories	134
Fat	4 g
Carbohydrate	27 g
Fiber	5 g
Protein	2 g
Calcium	111 mg
Iron	1.6 mg

Stuffed Zucchini

Makes 4 servings

Zucchini, a variety of summer squash, has a light, delicate flavor that is enhanced by the garlic-and-herb stuffing in this recipe. (And the stuffing is delicious with tomatoes, too!)

- **Preheat oven to 350°F (180°C)**
- **8-inch (20 cm) square glass baking dish, lightly greased**

2	zucchini	2
1	clove garlic, minced	1
¼ cup	gluten-free dry bread crumbs or cracker crumbs	60 mL
1 tbsp	chopped fresh parsley	15 mL
2 tsp	olive oil	10 mL
	Salt and freshly ground black pepper	

1. Cut off ends of zucchini, then cut zucchini in half lengthwise. Using a spoon, remove some of the flesh from the center of each zucchini half. Place cut side up in prepared baking dish.

2. In a small bowl, combine garlic, bread crumbs, parsley and oil. Season to taste with salt and pepper. Spread evenly in hollowed-out zucchini.

3. Cover and bake in preheated oven for 20 to 30 minutes or until zucchini are tender.

Variation

Substitute 2 large tomatoes for the zucchini and cook for 20 to 30 minutes or until tomatoes are tender.

Nutrients per serving

Calories	60
Fat	4 g
Carbohydrate	7 g
Fiber	1 g
Protein	1 g
Calcium	21 mg
Iron	0.5 mg

Roasted Root Veggies

Makes 4 servings

Nutrients per serving

Calories	103
Fat	7 g
Carbohydrate	10 g
Fiber	3 g
Protein	1 g
Calcium	37 mg
Iron	0.6 mg

- Preheat oven to 450°F (230°C)
- Large rimmed baking sheet

1 lb	root vegetables (such as parsnips, turnip, rutabaga, red, white or sweet potatoes, carrots, onions and beets)	500 g
2 tbsp	olive oil	30 mL
1 to 2	cloves garlic, minced	1 to 2
	Salt and freshly ground black pepper	

1. Peel and cut vegetables into bite-size chunks. In a large bowl or plastic bag (see tip, page 256), toss vegetables with oil and garlic. Lightly season with salt and pepper. Arrange on baking sheet in a single layer.

2. Roast in preheated oven, turning partway through, for 30 minutes or until tender and golden brown.

Fragrant Coconut Rice

Makes 4 servings

This is a deliciously rich rice.

Nutrients per serving

Calories	339
Fat	19 g
Carbohydrate	39 g
Fiber	4 g
Protein	5 g
Calcium	19 mg
Iron	3.7 mg

1½ cups	coconut milk	375 mL
1 cup	water	250 mL
1	2-inch (5 cm) cinnamon stick	1
1 cup	brown basmati or brown long-grain rice, rinsed and drained	250 mL

1. In a saucepan over medium-high heat, bring coconut milk, water and cinnamon stick to a rapid boil. Stir in rice and return to a boil. Reduce heat to low. Cover and simmer until rice is tender and liquid is absorbed, about 50 minutes.

Basmati Rice with Ginger

If plain rice tastes like cardboard because of reduced taste sensitivity, this recipe should hold some appeal for your damaged taste buds.

Make Ahead

Transfer cooked rice to individual shallow airtight containers and refrigerate for up to 2 days or freeze for up to 2 months. If frozen, thaw in the microwave or refrigerator. Reheat individual portions in the microwave on Medium-High (70%) for 2 to 3 minutes, or in a saucepan over medium heat, stirring often and adding a little water as necessary to moisten, for 3 to 4 minutes or until very hot.

Nutrients per serving

Calories	167
Fat	4 g
Carbohydrate	33 g
Fiber	2 g
Protein	3 g
Calcium	8 mg
Iron	0.8 mg

1½ cups	basmati rice	375 mL
1 tbsp	olive oil	15 mL
1	small onion, finely chopped	1
1 tbsp	minced gingerroot	15 mL
1	4-inch (10 cm) cinnamon stick, broken in half	1
1	large bay leaf, broken in half	1
1 tsp	salt	5 mL
2¼ cups	water	550 mL
¼ cup	chopped fresh cilantro (or 2 tbsp/30 mL chives or green onions)	60 mL

1. Place rice in sieve and rinse. Transfer to a bowl and add water to cover. Let soak for 15 minutes. Drain.

2. In a medium saucepan, heat oil over medium heat. Add onion, ginger, cinnamon and bay leaf; cook, stirring, for 2 minutes or until onion is softened.

3. Add rice, salt and water; bring to a boil. Reduce heat to low, cover and simmer for 10 minutes or until water is absorbed. Let stand, covered, for 5 minutes.

4. Fluff rice with a fork and remove and discard cinnamon stick and bay leaf. Serve sprinkled with cilantro.

Variation

To boost the fiber content and increase the cancer-fighting properties of this recipe, use brown basmati rice, increase the water to 3¾ cups (925 mL) and increase the cooking time to 30 minutes.

Quinoa Pilaf

Meet your new go-to side dish. This easy dish is endlessly versatile: vary the nuts and herbs, stir in leftover roasted or grilled vegetables, or add a touch of sweetness with dried fruit. You can even transform it into a main dish simply by adding your favorite protein, from cooked beans to grilled meat to canned tuna.

Tip

If using ready-to-use broth for this recipe, make sure to purchase one that is gluten-free.

1 cup	white, red or black quinoa, rinsed	250 mL
2 cups	Chicken Stock (page 179), Vegetable Stock (page 178) or reduced-sodium ready-to-use chicken or vegetable broth	500 mL
1 tbsp	extra virgin olive oil	15 mL
1¼ cups	chopped onions	300 mL
1	clove garlic, minced	1
½ cup	packed fresh flat-leaf (Italian) parsley leaves, chopped	125 mL
⅓ cup	lightly salted roasted almonds, chopped	75 mL
	Fine sea salt and freshly cracked black pepper	

1. In a medium saucepan, combine quinoa and stock. Bring to a boil over medium-high heat. Reduce heat to low, cover and simmer for 12 to 15 minutes or until liquid is absorbed. Remove from heat and let stand, covered, for 5 minutes. Fluff with a fork.

2. Meanwhile, in a large nonstick skillet, heat oil over medium-high heat. Add onions and cook, stirring, for 6 to 8 minutes or until softened. Add garlic and cook, stirring, for 1 minute. Add quinoa and cook, stirring, for 2 minutes. Remove from heat and stir in parsley and almonds. Season to taste with salt and pepper.

Nutrients per serving

Calories	286
Fat	11 g
Carbohydrate	37 g
Fiber	6 g
Protein	12 g
Calcium	80 mg
Iron	3.2 mg

Desserts

Macerated Berries

Makes 2 servings

Here's a simple and easy technique for softening berries. This dessert is quick to make and can be prepared ahead of time and refrigerated until you're ready to eat.

Tip

Substitute any soft berry for those called for in this recipe, so long as the total amount adds up to 1½ cups (375 mL). You can add finely grated lemon zest as well.

1 cup	sliced hulled strawberries (about ½ pint)	250 mL
¼ cup	blueberries	60 mL
¼ cup	blackberries	60 mL
3 tbsp	raw agave nectar	45 mL
2 tbsp	freshly squeezed lemon juice	30 mL
Dash	raw vanilla extract	Dash

1. In a bowl, toss strawberries, blueberries, blackberries, agave nectar, lemon juice and vanilla. Set aside for 30 to 45 minutes or until berries are soft and liquid is seeping out of the fruit. Serve immediately or cover and refrigerate for up to 3 days.

Nutrients per serving

Calories	137
Fat	0 g
Carbohydrate	35 g
Fiber	3 g
Protein	1 g
Calcium	19 mg
Iron	0.5 mg

Avocado Lemon Curd

Makes 4 servings

This slightly sweet yet pleasantly tangy dessert melts in your mouth.

Tips

Coconut butter is a blend of coconut oil and coconut meat that is high in healthy fats and adds creaminess to smoothies and sauces. It is available in the nut butter section of natural foods stores or well-stocked supermarkets.

Coconut oil is solid at room temperature. It has a melting temperature of 76°F (24°C), so it is easy to liquefy. Place the required amount in a shallow glass bowl and place the bowl over a pot of simmering water.

Nutrients per serving	
Calories	399
Fat	32 g
Carbohydrate	30 g
Fiber	5 g
Protein	4 g
Calcium	35 mg
Iron	0.8 mg

- Blender
- Four ½-cup (125 mL) ramekins

2 tsp	finely grated lemon zest	10 mL
⅓ cup	freshly squeezed lemon juice	75 mL
⅓ cup	raw agave nectar	75 mL
¼ cup	chopped avocado	60 mL
¼ cup	coconut butter (see tip, at left)	60 mL
¼ cup	melted coconut oil (see tip, at left)	60 mL
2 tbsp	almond butter	30 mL
2 tbsp	cashew butter	30 mL

1. In blender, combine lemon zest and juice, agave nectar, avocado and coconut butter. Blend until smooth and creamy. Add coconut oil, almond butter and cashew butter and blend until smooth.

2. Transfer to ramekins and refrigerate for at least 2 hours or up to 3 days. When you're ready to serve, remove from molds and serve.

Mango and Ginger Cashew Mousse

Makes 4 servings

This light and creamy mousse pairs particularly well with tropical fruits.

Tip

To soak the cashews for this recipe, place in a bowl and add 2 cups (500 mL) water. Cover and set aside for 30 minutes. Drain, discarding soaking water, and rinse under cold running water until the water runs clear.

• Blender

1 cup	raw cashews, soaked (see tip, at left)	250 mL
1 cup	chopped mango	250 mL
1/4 cup	filtered water	60 mL
3 tbsp	raw agave nectar	45 mL
2 tbsp	chopped gingerroot	30 mL
2 tsp	freshly squeezed lemon juice	10 mL

1. In blender, combine soaked cashews, mango, water, agave nectar, ginger and lemon juice. Blend at high speed until smooth and creamy.

Variation

For a slightly tarter version of this mousse, substitute $1/2$ cup (125 mL) chopped pineapple and $1/4$ cup (60 mL) chopped peeled apple for the mango.

Nutrients per serving

Calories	252
Fat	14 g
Carbohydrate	29 g
Fiber	2 g
Protein	6 g
Calcium	18 mg
Iron	2.3 mg

Lemon Avocado Mousse

This dessert has a creamy, smooth, pudding-like consistency that melts in the mouth.

Tip

To use the flesh of a lemon, place on a cutting board and cut slices from the top and bottom to create flat surfaces. Using a sharp knife in a downward motion, remove the skin and the pith. Shave off any remaining bits of pith, then cut between the membranes to produce wedges of pure citrus flesh.

Nutrients per serving

Calories	305
Fat	11 g
Carbohydrate	56 g
Fiber	5 g
Protein	2 g
Calcium	11 mg
Iron	0.5 mg

• **Food processor**

2 cups	chopped avocado	500 mL
½ cup	freshly squeezed lemon juice	125 mL
¼ cup	lemon segments (see tip, at left)	60 mL
¾ cup	raw agave nectar	175 mL

1. In food processor, process avocado, lemon juice and lemon segments until smooth, stopping the motor and scraping down the sides of the work bowl as necessary. With the motor running, drizzle agave nectar through the feed tube, combining well.

2. Serve immediately or transfer to an airtight container and refrigerate for up to 3 days.

Cashew Whipped Cream

This cream is light and fluffy and tastes just as delicious as the dairy version. It is a perfect finish for Macerated Berries (page 262), among other desserts.

Tips

To soak the cashews for this recipe, place in a bowl and add 4 cups (1 L) water. Cover and set aside for 30 minutes. Drain, discarding soaking water, and rinse under cold running water until the water runs clear.

If you have a high-powered blender, use it to make this cream. It will be smoother and creamier than when made in a regular blender.

Nutrients per ¼ cup (60 mL)

Calories	138
Fat	8 g
Carbohydrate	15 g
Fiber	1 g
Protein	3 g
Calcium	7 mg
Iron	1.2 mg

• Blender

2 cups	raw cashews, soaked (see tip, at left)	500 mL
1 cup	filtered water	250 mL
½ cup	raw agave nectar	125 mL
1 tsp	vanilla extract	5 mL
¼ tsp	freshly squeezed lemon juice	1 mL

1. In blender, combine soaked cashews, water, agave nectar, vanilla and lemon juice. Blend at high speed until smooth and creamy. Transfer to a bowl, cover and refrigerate for up to 5 days.

Variations

Vanilla Pine Nut Whipped Cream: Substitute 2 cups (500 mL) pine nuts for the cashews.

Brazil Nut Whipped Cream: Substitute 2 cups (500 mL) Brazil nuts for the cashews.

Pineapple Lime Sorbet

This light, refreshing dessert satisfies your sweet tooth without leaving you feeling heavy.

Tip

To make 1¼ cups (300 mL) puréed pineapple, you will need a fresh pineapple weighing about 1½ lbs (750 g). Peel and core it and cut it into chunks, then blend at medium speed until smooth. You can also use pineapple canned in juice. About 1¾ cups (425 mL) drained pineapple chunks will make 1¼ cups (300 mL) purée.

• **Ice cream maker**

1¼ cups	pineapple purée	300 mL
2 tsp	grated lime or lemon zest	10 mL
¾ cup	freshly squeezed lime or lemon juice	175 mL
¼ cup	water	60 mL
	Thin slices lime or lemon	

1. In a bowl, stir together pineapple purée, lime zest, lime juice and water.

2. In ice cream maker, freeze according to manufacturer's directions.

3. Divide among four individual dessert dishes. Serve garnished with thin slice of lime.

Nutrients per serving

Calories	60
Fat	0 g
Carbohydrate	17 g
Fiber	1 g
Protein	1 g
Calcium	15 mg
Iron	0.1 mg

Raspberry Ice with Fresh Strawberries

Fruity and refreshing, this icy treat is also full of antioxidants — perfect for a hot summer day!

- **Blender or food processor**
- **Ice cream maker**

4½ cups	fresh raspberries	1.125 L
	Honey	
6	large fresh strawberries	6
	Fresh mint leaves	

1. In blender, purée raspberries. Strain to remove seeds. Stir in honey to taste.

2. In ice cream maker, freeze according to manufacturer's directions.

3. Divide among six individual dessert dishes. Garnish each serving with a strawberry and mint leaves.

Peach Granita

You'll love this cool and refreshing source of vitamin C.

Tip

If using pure cranberry juice, taste and add liquid honey, brown rice syrup or agave nectar to sweeten.

• **Blender**

1 cup	cranberry juice	250 mL
4	ice cubes	4
1 cup	frozen peach slices	250 mL

1. In blender, combine cranberry juice, ice cubes and peaches. Secure lid and process using the chop or pulse function until smooth. Serve immediately with a spoon.

Nutrients per serving	
Calories	176
Fat	1 g
Carbohydrate	46 g
Fiber	3 g
Protein	2 g
Calcium	30 mg
Iron	1.0 mg

Watermelon-Strawberry Splash

What better way to make a splash than with this antioxidant-rich combination?

• **Blender**

½ cup	raspberry or cranberry juice	125 mL
2 tbsp	freshly squeezed lemon juice	30 mL
1 cup	chopped watermelon	250 mL
6	frozen strawberries	6

1. In blender, combine raspberry juice, lemon juice, watermelon and strawberries. Secure lid and blend (from low to high if using a variable-speed blender) until smooth.

Nutrients per serving

Calories	70
Fat	0 g
Carbohydrate	20 g
Fiber	2 g
Protein	1 g
Calcium	20 mg
Iron	0.6 mg

Tart and Tingly Smoothie

Blueberries are an excellent antioxidant. Tantalize your taste buds with this sweet-tart blend that's rich in vitamin C.

Tips

Some people have an adverse reaction to raw elderberries. If in doubt, cook, cool and drain before using.

You can use fresh and frozen fruit interchangeably in most smoothies, although the results will differ. Frozen fruit not only chills a smoothie, it thickens it as well.

• **Blender**

¼ cup	cranberry juice	60 mL
2	kiwifruit, quartered	2
½ cup	frozen blueberries or elderberries (see tip, at left)	125 mL
	Honey (optional)	

1. In blender, combine cranberry juice, kiwis and blueberries. Secure lid and blend (from low to high if using a variable-speed blender) until smooth. Pour into a glass and stir in honey to taste, if desired.

Nutrients per serving	
Calories	148
Fat	1 g
Carbohydrate	37 g
Fiber	6 g
Protein	2 g
Calcium	52 mg
Iron	0.6 mg

Pomegranate Perfect

This refreshing combination is both nutritious and delicious! It is rich in antioxidants and immune-supportive nutrients, including vitamin C.

Tip

Among its many benefits, coconut milk is high in manganese (important for blood sugar regulation) and phosphorus (important for bone health).

- **Blender**

½ cup	coconut milk	125 mL
1	slice watermelon, cut into chunks	1
½ cup	raspberries	125 mL
¼ cup	pomegranate seeds	60 mL

1. In blender, combine coconut milk, watermelon, raspberries and pomegranate seeds. Secure lid and blend (from low to high if using a variable-speed blender) until smooth.

Nutrients per serving

Calories	383
Fat	29 g
Carbohydrate	35 g
Fiber	5 g
Protein	5 g
Calcium	44 mg
Iron	2.6 mg

Contributing Authors

Alexandra Anca with
Theresa Santandrea-Cull
Complete Gluten-Free Diet & Nutrition Guide
Recipes from this book are found on pages 193, 195, 222 (top), 242, 251 and 257.

Byron Ayanoglu with
contributions from Algis Kemezys
125 Best Vegetarian Recipes
A recipe from this book is found on page 248.

Byron Ayanoglu and Jennifer MacKenzie
Complete Curry Cookbook
Recipes from this book are found on pages 190 and 232.

Johanna Burkhard
500 Best Comfort Food Recipes
A recipe from this book is found on page 259.

Johanna Burkhard
Diabetes Comfort Food
A recipe from this book is found on page 169.

Andrew Chase and Nicole Young
The Blender Bible
A recipe from this book is found on page 170.

Pat Crocker
The Smoothies Bible, 2nd edition
Recipes from this book are found on pages 174–76 and 269–72.

Pat Crocker
The Vegetarian Cook's Bible
A recipe from this book is found on page 208.

Dietitians of Canada
Cook Great Food
Recipes from this book are found on pages 224, 244 and 253.

Dietitians of Canada
Simply Great Food
Recipes from this book are found on pages 218, 223, 237 and 240.

Judith Finlayson
The Complete Whole Grains Cookbook
Recipes from this book are found on pages 163, 165, 198 and 258 (bottom).

Judith Finlayson
The Convenience Cook
A recipe from this book is found on page 196.

Judith Finlayson
The Healthy Slow Cooker
Recipes from this book are found on pages 164, 182, 188 and 230.

Judith Finlayson
The Vegetarian Slow Cooker
Recipes from this book are found on pages 185 and 229.

George Geary and Judith Finlayson
650 Best Food Processor Recipes
A recipe from this book is found on page 205.

Margaret Howard
The 250 Best 4-Ingredient Recipes
Recipes from this book are found on pages 194, 214 (top), 215 (top), 220, 234, 236, 238–39, 243, 246, 249, 255–56 and 258 (top).

Douglas McNish
Eat Raw, Eat Well
Recipes from this book are found on pages 202–4, 207, 214 (bottom), 215 (bottom), 216 and 262–266.

Dr. Maitreyi Raman, Angela Sirounis
and Jennifer Shrubsole
The Complete IBS Health & Diet Guide
A recipe from this book is found on page 222 (bottom).

Lynn Roblin, Nutrition Editor
500 Best Healthy Recipes
Recipes from this book are found on pages 178, 179, 267 and 268.

Deb Roussou
350 Best Vegan Recipes
A recipe from this book is found on page 206.

Camilla V. Saulsbury
5 Easy Steps to Healthy Cooking
Recipes from this book are found on pages 162, 168, 173, 180, 211, 219, 221, 227, 228, 241, 250, 252 and 254.

Camilla V. Saulsbury
500 Best Quinoa Recipes
Recipes from this book are found on pages 166, 167, 171, 172, 181, 184, 186, 189, 192, 197, 210, 212, 213, 225, 233, 245 and 260.

Mary Sue Waisman
Dietitians of Canada Cook!
Recipes from this book are found on pages 200 and 226.

Resources

Chief Resources

American Association of Naturopathic Physicians: www.naturopathic.org

Bested, Alison C, et al. *Hope and Help for Chronic Fatigue Syndrome and Fibromyalgia*. Nashville, TN: Cumberland House, 2008.

Canadian Association of Naturopathic Doctors: www.cand.ca

Fibromylagia Association UK: www.fibromyalgia-associationuk.org

Glycemic Index: www.glycemicindex.com

Guided imagery CDs by Belleruth Naparstek: www.belleruthnaparstek.com

Harvard Mind-Body Medical Institute programs: www.mbmi.org

ME/FM Action Network: www.mefmaction.net

National Chronic Fatigue Syndrome and Fibromyalgia Association: www.ncfsfs.org

National Fibromyalgia and Chronic Pain Association: www.fmcpaware.org

National Fibromyalgia Association/*Fibromyalgia AWARE* magazine: www.fmaware.org

National Fibromyalgia Research Association: www.nfra.net

Nelson, Miriam. *Strong Women Stay Young*. New York, NY: Bantam Books, 1997.

Associations and Agencies

National Fibromyalgia Association

The NFA has worked since 1997 to provide support for people with fibromyalgia and other chronic pain illnesses. The association hosts international conferences, puts on National Fibromyalgia Awareness Week, and publishes *Fibromyalgia AWARE* magazine.

International Association for CFS/ME

A nonprofit organization that emphasizes research, patient care, and treatment. It conducts international scientific conferences to promote and evaluate research, and looks for ways to use research to help doctors and patients. Noted ME/CFS researcher Nancy Klimas, MD, is currently president.

CFIDS Association of America

A charitable organization that aims to bring an end to the suffering and disability caused by chronic fatigue syndrome. Founded in 1987, it works to get federal funding for research, make Social Security disability funds more accessible to people with ME/CFS, educate doctors, and provide reliable information.

National Fibromyalgia Research Association

A nonprofit organization that helps fund research and education, raise public awareness, and lobby the government to get more funding for research and recognition. This group has also created a fibromyalgia awareness bracelet and co-produced a fibromyalgia exercise video.

American Fibromyalgia Syndrome Association

A nonprofit group that funds research in fibromyalgia by providing pilot grants to help scientists persuade the government or other agencies to fund studies. Two prominent fibromyalgia researchers, Drs. Charles Lapp and Daniel Clauw, are on the association's Medical Advisory Committee.

H.O.P.E. — Helping Our Pain and Exhaustion

A nonprofit organization that works to educate friends and families, the public, the media, and the medical community about fibromyalgia and chronic fatigue syndrome. Leading researcher Daniel Clauw, MD, is on the group's advisory board.

American Pain Foundation

A nonprofit group that works to improve the quality of life of people living with pain through public awareness, promoting research, and removing barriers to effective pain management. The APF worked to support the National Pain Care Policy Act, which passed the U.S. House of Representatives in September 2008.

Rest Ministries

A nonprofit Christian organization with a focus on support and awareness. It publishes *Hopekeepers Magazine* and also founded National Invisible Chronic Illness Awareness Week.

Advocacy Groups

MEFM (Myalgic Encephalomyelitis and Fibromyalgia Societies of BC)
www.mefm.bc.ca
604-878-7707 or B.C. toll-free 1-888-353-6322

National ME/FM Action Network
www.mefmaction.net
613-829-6667

Fibromyalgia Support Group
www.mefm.bc.ca
604-944-2506

Fibromyalgia Wellspring Foundation
http://www.fibromyalgiawellspringfoundation
1-800-567-8998 or 604-530-4173

ME Victoria Association
http://members.shaw.ca/me/victoria
250-370-2884

ME/FM B.C. Speakers Forum www.f2c2.ca

ME/CFS and FM Support Group
www.mefmgroup.wordpress.com

Other Resources

Resources for living with fibromyalgia:
www.fibrocentre.ca

Tools for managing ME/FM: www.cfidsselfhelp.org

ME/FM online self-study course:
www.treatcfsfm.org/index.html

ME/CFS and FM Support Group:
www.mefmgroup.wordpress.com

Fibromyalgia online self-study course:
www.trentcfsfm.org/index.html

Self-management program: www.fibroguide.com

Practical tools for managing fibromyalgia:
www.cfidsselfhelp.org

Women's health and living with ME/CFS:
www.womenshealthmatters.ca/health-resources/
environmental-health/chronic-fatigue-syndrome/
medical-description

Vancouver Coastal Health: www.vch.ca/locations_
and_services/find_health_services

Dr. Mike Evans, Health Topics:
www.myfavouritemedicine.com

Related Resources

Pain Management
Canadian Pain Society
www.canadianpainsociety.ca
Advocates for women's health, offers resources for managing pain and operates the Canadian Pain Coalition.

Pain B.C.
www.painbc.ca
Offers webinars, workshops, and the Pain Toolbox to encourage prevention and early intervention of chronic pain.

Pain Toolkit
www.pipain.com
An information booklet offered by the People in Pain Network. Provides tips for managing pain.

Pain Self-Management Program
www.selfmanage.org/onlinebc or
www.coag.uvic.ca/cdsmp
Free 6-week online workshop and in-person peer support to help manage chronic pain.

Disability Resources
B.C. Coalition for Persons with Disabilities
www.bccpd.bc.ca
604-872-1278 or 1-800-663-1278
Helps people with disabilities live with dignity and independence. Provides the Disability/CPP forms guide.

Disabilities Resource Guide
www.oftdf.org
Provides information, education, and employment resources for people with disabilities. Promotes accessible transportation.

Legal Assistance
B.C. Law Students' Legal Advice Program
www.lslap.bc.ca
604-822-5791

B.C. Click Law
www.clicklaw.bc.ca

Legal Aid B.C.
www.legalaid.bc.ca
1-866-577-2525

Diet and Nutrition
Canada's Food Guide: http://hc-sc.gc.ca/fn-an/
food-guide-aliment/index-eng.php

USDA MyPlate food guide: www.choosemyplate.gov

Harvest Box Program
www.fraservalleyfoodnetwork.com
778-228-6614
Low-cost fresh produce for families in Delta, Surrey, White Rock, and Langley, B.C.

Physiotherapy
Canadian Physiotherapy Association:
www.physiotherapy.ca

American Physical Therapy Association:
www.apta.org

B.C. Physiotherapy Directory: www.bcphysio.org

References

Agricultural Research Service (ARS) Nutrient Database for Standard Reference, Release 17.

Akkaya N, et al. Assessment of the relationship between postural stability and sleep quality in patients with fibromyalgia. Clin Rheumatol. 2013;32(3):325–31.

Ardic F, Ozgen M, Aybek H, et al. Effects of balneotherapy on serum IL-1, PGE2 and LTB4 levels in fibromyalgia patients. Rheumatol Int. 2007;27:441–46.

Arnold LM, et al. Family study of fibromyalgia. Arthritis Rheum. 2004;50:944–52. Other research has shown the genes that help modulate pain in the brain may also be involved: COMT, dopamine receptor, serotonin transporter and 5-HT receptor genes.

Arnold LM, Fan J, Russell IJ, Yunus MB, Khan MA, Kushner I, Olson JM, Iyengar SK. The fibromyalgia family study: A genome-scan linkage study. Arthritis Rheum. 2012 Dec 28. doi: 10.1002/art.37842 [Epub ahead of print].

Ather Ali ND, et. al. Intravenous micronutrient therapy (Myers' Cocktail) for fibromyalgia: A placebo-controlled pilot study. J Altern Complement Med. 2009 March;15(3): 247–57.

Atzeni F, et al. The evaluation of the fibromyalgia patients. Reumatismo (Journal of Italian Society for Rheumatology). 2008;60(1):36–49.

Baranowsky J, et al. Qualitative systemic review of randomized controlled trials on complementary and alternative medicine treatments in fibromyalgia. Rheumatol Int. 2009;30(1):1–21.

Bazzichi L, et al. Altered amino acid homeostasis in subjects affected by fibromyalgia. Clin Biochem. 2009;42(10–11): 1064–70.

Behm FG, et al. Unique immunologic patterns in fibromyalgia. BMC Clinical Pathology. 2012;12:25.

Bell IR, Lewis DA 2nd, Brooks AJ, Schwartz GE, Lewis SE, Walsh BT, Baldwin CM. Improved clinical status in fibromyalgia patients treated with individualized homeopathic remedies versus placebo. Rheumatology (Oxford). 2004 May;43(5):577–82.

Bent S, Patterson M, Garvin D. Valerian for sleep: A systematic review and meta-analysis. Altern Therapies. 2001;7:S4.

Bondy B, et al. 5-HTP2A receptor polymorphism in fibromyalgia. Neurobiol Dis. 1999;6:433–39.

Bote ME, et al. Inflammatory/stress feedback dysregulation in women with fibromyalgia. Neuroimmunomodulation. 2012;19(6):343–51.

Boyle W, Saine A. Lectures in Naturopathic Hydrotherapy. Eclectic Medical Publications;2001.

Brattberg G. Connective tissue massage in the treatment of fibromyalgia. Eur J Pain. 1999 Jun;3(3): 235–44.

Brummett CM, Clauw DJ. Fibromyalgia: A primer for the anesthesia community. Curr Opin Anaesthesiol. 2011;24(5):532–39.

Brzezinski A. Melatonin in humans. N Engl J Med 1997;336:186–95.

Buskila D, et al. An association between fibromyalgia and the dopamine D4 receptor exon III repeat polymorphism and relationship to novelty seeking personality traits. Mol Psychiatry. 2004;9:730–31.

Buskila D, Abu-Shakra M, Neumann L, et al. Balneotherapy for fibromyalgia at the Dead Sea. Rheumatol Int. 2001;20: 105–8.

Buskila D, Sarzi-Puttini P. Biology and therapy of fibromyalgia: Genetic aspects of fibromyalgia syndrome. Arthritis Res & Therapy. 2006;8:218–22.

Canadian Community Health Survey. 2010.

Cao H. Medicinal cupping therapy in 30 patients with fibromyalgia: A case series observation. H. Forschende Komplementarmedizin. 2011 Jun;18(3):122–26.

Caruso I, Sarzi Puttini P, Cazzola M, Azzolini V. Double-blind study of 5-hydroxytryptophan versus placebo in the treatment of primary fibromyalgia syndrome. J Int Med Res. 1990;18:201–9.

Castro-Sánchez AM, et al. A randomized controlled trial investigating the effects of craniosacral therapy on pain and heart rate variability in fibromyalgia patients. Clin Rehab. 2011 Jan;25(1): 25–35.

Cerny A, Shmid K. Tolerability and efficacy of valerian/lemon balm (a double blind, placebo-controlled, multicentre study). Fitoterapia. 1999;70:221–28.

Chen H. Fibromylagia with traditional Chinese medicine. Int J Clin Acupuncture. 2010 Oct;19(4):178–79.

Citera G, et al. The effect of melatonin in patients with fibromyalgia: A pilot study. Clin Rheumatol. 2000;19:9–13.

Connor WE. Importance of n-3 fatty acids in health and disease. Am J Clin Nutr. 2000;71:171S–75S.

Cordero MD, et al. 2012. Oral coenzyme Q10 supplementation improves clinical symptoms and recovers pathologic alterations in blood mononuclear cells in a fibromyalgia patient. Nutrition. 2012 Nov–Dec;28(11–12):1200–1203.

Cordero MD, Moreno-Fernandez AM, deMiguel M, et al. Coenzyme Q10 distribution in blood is altered in patients with fibromyalgia. Clin Biochem. 2009;42:732–35.

Curtis K, Osadchuk A, Katz J. An eight-week yoga intervention is associated with improvements in pain, psychological functioning and mindfulness, and changes in cortisol levels in women with fibromyalgia. J Pain Res. 2011;4:189–201.

Donath F, et al. Critical evaluation of the effect of valerian extract on sleep structure and sleep quality. Pharmacopsychiatry. 2000;33:47–53.

Duschek S, Werner NS, Winkelmann A, Wankner S. Implicit memory function in fibromyalgia syndrome. Behav Med. 2003 Jan;39(1):11–16.

Environmental Working Group Top Dirty and Clean Foods. www.ewg.org/foodnews/summary.

Evicik D, Kizilay B, Gokcen E. The effects of balneotherapy on fibromyalgia patients. Rheumatol Int. 2002;22:56–59.

Field T, et al. Fibromyalgia pain and substance P decreases and sleep improves following massage therapy. J Clin Rheumatol. 2002 Apr;8(2):72–76.

File SE, Fluck E, Fernandes C. Beneficial effects of glycine (bioglycin) on memory and attention in young and middle-aged adults. J Clin Psychopharmacol. 1999;19:506–12.

Fitzcharles M-A, et al. 2012 Canadian guidelines for the diagnosis and management of fibromyalgia syndrome. http://fmguidelines.ca.

Fitzcharles M-A, Peter A. Ste-Marie, Don L. Goldenberg, John X. Frequency. J Altern Complement Med. 2005 Aug; lino. 4: 665–71.

Friedlander JI, Shorter B, Moldwin RM. Diet and its role in interstitial cystitis/bladder pain syndrome (IC/BPS) and comorbid conditions. BJU Int. 2012 Jun;109(11):1584–91.

Gamber RG, Shores JH, Russo DP, Jimenez C, Rubin BR. Osteopathic manipulative treatment in conjunction with medication relieves pain associated with fibromyalgia syndrome: Results of a randomized clinical pilot project. J Am Osteopath Assoc. 2002 Jun;102(6):321–25.

Garcia-Fructuoso F, et al. Work by Arnold shows an increased risk with first degree relatives to have fibromyalgia. Barcelona Spain, IACFS Conference, Jan. 2007.

Glombiewski JA, et al. Psychological treatments for fibromyalgia: A meta-analysis. Pain. 2010;151(2):280–95.

Gonzalez B, et al. Fibromyalgia: Antecedent life events, disability, and causal attribution. Psychol Health Med. 2013; Jan 17 [Epub].

Gracely RH, Ambrose, KR. Neuroimaging of fibromyalgia. Best P&R Clin Rheumatol. 2011;25(2):271–84.

Gracely RH, et al. Functional magnetic resonance imaging evidence of augmented pain processing in fibromyalgia. Arth & Rheum. 2002;46(5):1333–43.

Gursoy S, et al. COMPT gene polymorphism. Rheumatol Int. 2003;104–7.

Hadianfard MJ, Hosseinzadeh Parizi M. A randomized clinical trial of fibromyalgia treatment with acupuncture compared with fluoxetine. Iran Red Crescent Med J. 2012 Oct;14(10):631–40.

Harris RE, et al. Treatment of fibromyalgia with formula acupuncture: Investigation of needle placement, needle stimulation, and treatment. J Altern Complement Med. 2005 Aug;11(4):663–71.

Harris R, et al. Decreased central μ-opioid receptor availability in fibromyalgia. J Neuroscience. 2007;27(37): 10000–6.

Hoffer A and Prousky J. Naturopathic Nutrition: A Guide to Nutrient-Rich Food & Nutritional Supplements for Optimal Health. Toronto, ON:CCNM Press, 2006.

Hsu MC, et al. Sustained pain reduction through affective self-awareness in fibromyalgia: A randomized controlled trial. J Gen Intern Med. 2010 Oct;25(10):1064–70.

International Table of Glycemic Index and Load Values: 2002. Am J Clin Nutr. 2002;62:5–56.

International Tables of Glycemic Index and Glycemic Load Values: 2008. Fiona S. Atkinson, RD, Kaye Foster-Powell, RD, Jennie C. Brand-Miller, PhD. http://care.diabetesjournals.org.

Izquierdo-Alvarez S, et al. Is there an association between fibromyalgia and below-normal levels of urinary cortisol? BMC Res Notes. 2008;22(1):134.

Jacobsen S, Danneskiold-Samsoe B, Andersen RB. Oral S-adenosylmethionine in primary fibromyalgia: Double-blind clinical evaluation. Scand J Rheumatol 1991;20:294–302.

Jain A, et al. Fibromyalgia syndrome: Canadian clinical working case definition, diagnostic and treatment protocols — a consensus document. J Musculoskeletal Pain. 2009; 11(4):3–107.

Jensen KB, et al. Patients with fibromyalgia display less functional connectivity in the brain's pain inhibitory network. Mol Pain. 2012 Apr 26;8:32.

Jones GT, et al. Role of road traffic accidents and other traumatic events in the onset of chronic widespread pain: Results from a population-based prospective study. Arthritis Care Res (Hoboken). 2011;63(5):696–701.

Khalsa KP. Bodywork for fibromyalgia: Alternative therapies soothe the pain. Massage Bodywork. 2009 May 1;24(3): 80–89.

Kim SH, et al. Insular cortex is a trait marker for pain processing in fibromyalgia syndrome-blood oxygenation level-dependent functional magnetic resonance imaging study in Korea. Clin Exp Rheumatol. 2011;29(6 Suppl 69):S19–S27.

Kishi A, et al. Sleep-stage dynamics in patients with chronic fatigue syndrome with or without fibromyalgia. Sleep. 2011 Nov 1;34(11):1551–60.

Klepser TB, Klepser ME. Unsafe and potentially safe herbal therapies. Am J Health Syst Pharm. 1999;56:125–38.

Kuptniratsaikul V, et al. Efficacy and safety of Curcuma domestica extracts in patients with knee osteoarthritis. J Altern Complement Med. 2009;15:891–97.

Lawrence RC, et al. Estimates of the prevalence of arthritis and other rheumatic conditions in the United States. Part II. Arthritis Rheum. 2008;58(1):26–35.

Liew CV, et al. Predictors of pain and functioning over time in fibromyalgia syndrome: An autoregressive path analysis. Arthritis Care Res. 2013;65(2):251–56.

Light AR, et al. Gene expression alterations at baseline and following moderate exercise in patients with chronic fatigue syndrome, and fibromyalgia syndrome. J Intern Med. 2012; 271(1):64–81.

Lister RE. An open, pilot study to evaluate the potential benefits of coenzyme Q10 combined with Ginkgo biloba extract in fibromyalgia syndrome. J Int Med Res. 2002;30:195–99.

Marcus DA, et al. Fibromyalgia family and relationship impact exploratory survey. Musculoskeletal Care. 2012;21 [Epub].

Martínez-Jauand M, et al. Age-of-onset of menopause is associated with enhanced painful and non-painful sensitivity in fibromyalgia. Clin Rheumatol. 2013 Feb 16 [Epub].

Martínez-Jauand M, et al. Pain sensitivity in fibromyalgia is associated with catechol-O-methyltransferase (COMT) gene. Eur J Pain. 2013;17(1):16–27.

Marz RB. Medical Nutrition from Marz. 2nd ed. Portland, OR: Omnivite Nutrition, 2010.

McCarty DJ, et al. Treatment of pain due to fibromyalgia with topical capsaicin: A pilot study. Semin Arthr Rheum 1994;23:41–47.

Mishra LC, Singh BB, Dagenais S. Scientific basis for the therapeutic use of Withania somnifera (ashwagandha): A review. Altern Med Rev. 2000;5:334–46.

Moldofsky H, et al. Effects of bedtime very low dose cyclobenzaprine on symptoms and sleep physiology in patients with fibromyalgia syndrome: A double-blind randomized placebo-controlled study. J Rheumatol. 2011;38(12):2653–63.

National ME/FM Action Network, from the Statistics Canada data file for the 2005 Canadian Community Health Survey.

Newberg AB, et al. Double-blind, placebo-controlled, randomized pilot study of cerebral blood flow patterns employing SPECT imaging in dental postsurgical pain patients with and without pain relief. Clin Therapeutics. 2011;33(12):1894–1903.

Ngan A, Conduit R. A double-blind, placebo-controlled investigation of the effects of Passiflora incarnata (passionflower) herbal tea on subjective sleep quality. Phytother Res. 2011;25:1153–59.

Nicolodi M, Sicuteri F. Fibromyalgia and migraine, two faces of the same mechanism: Serotonin as the common clue for pathogenesis and therapy. Adv Exp Med Biol. 1996;398: 373–79.

Okifuji A, et al. Relationship between fibromyalgia and obesity in pain, function, mood and sleep. J Pain. 2010;11(12):1329–37.

Parlor M. Quest Newsletter #88, Summer 2011. National ME/FM Action Network. www.mefmaction.com.

Pauer L, et al. An international, randomized, double-blind, placebo-controlled, phase III trial of pregabalin monotherapy in treatment of patients with fibromyalgia. J Rheumatol. 2011;38(12):2643–52.

Paul-Savoie E, et al. Is the deficit in pain inhibition in fibromyalgia influenced by sleep impairments? Open Rheumatol J. 2012;6:296–302.

Pérez-de-Heredia-Torres M, et al. Bilateral deficits in fine motor control ability and manual dexterity in women with fibromyalgia syndrome. Exp Brain Res. 2013 Jan 26 [Epub].

Prousky JE. Mild adrenocortical deficiency and its relationship to: (1) Chronic Fatigue Syndrome; (2) Nausea and Vomiting of Pregnancy and Hyperemesis Gravidarum; and (3) Systemic Lupus Erythematosus. J Orthomolecular Med. 2012;27(4):165–76.

Pureti MB, Demarin V. Neuroplasticity mechanisms in the pathophysiology of chronic pain. Acta Clin Croat. 2012 Sep;51(3):425–29. Review.

Reeser JC, et al. Apolipoprotein e4 genotype increases the risk of being diagnosed with posttraumatic fibromyalgia. PM R. 2011;3(3):193–97.

Russell IJ, Michalek JE, Flechas JD, Abraham GE. Treatment of fibromyalgia syndrome with Super Malic: A randomized, double blind, placebo controlled, crossover pilot study. J Rheumatol. 1995 May;22(5):953–58.

Sarzi Puttini P, Caruso I. Primary fibromyalgia syndrome and 5-hydroxy-L-tryptophan: A 90-day open study. J Int Med Res. 1992;20:182–89.

Schmidt S, et al. Treating fibromyalgia with mindfulness-based stress reduction: Results from a 3-armed randomized controlled trial. Pain. 2011;152(2):361–69.

Shevtsov VA, et al. A randomized trial of two different doses of a SHR-5 Rhodiola rosea extract versus placebo and control of capacity for mental work. Phytomedicine. 2003;10:95–105.

Simopoulos AP, Leaf A, Salem N. Workshop statement on the essentiality of and recommended dietary intakes for omega-6 and omega-3 fatty acids. Prostaglandins. Leukot Essent Fatty Acids. 2000;63:119–21.

Sukenik S, et al. Balneotherapy at the Dead Sea area for patients with psoriatic arthritis and concommitant fibromyalgia. Isr Med Assoc J. 2001;3:147–50.

Tavoni A, Vitali C, Bombardieri S, Pasero G. Evaluation of S-adenosylmethionine in primary fibromyalgia: A double-blind crossover study. Am J Med. 1987;83:107–10.

Teitelbaum JE, Johnson C, St Cyr J. The use of D-ribose in chronic fatigue syndrome and fibromyalgia: A pilot study. J Altern Complement Med. 2006;12:857–62.

Toussaint L, et al. A mind-body technique (amygdala retraining) for symptoms related to fibromyalgia and chronic fatigue. Explore (NY). 2012;8(2):92–98.

Upton R, ed. Ashwagandha root (Withania somnifera): Analytical, quality control, and therapeutic monograph. Santa Cruz, CA: American Herbal Pharmacopoeia, 2000:1–25.

Veldhuijzen DS, et al. Intact cognitive inhibition in patients with fibromyalgia but evidence of declined processing speed. J Pain. 2012;13(5):507–15.

Vincent A, Lahr BD, Wolfe F, et al. Prevalence of fibromyalgia: A population-based study in Olmsted County, Minnesota, utilizing the Rochester Epidemiology project. Arthritis Care Res (Hoboken). 2012 Nov 30. doi: 10.1002/acr.21896 [Epub ahead of print].

Wagner JS, et al. The association of sleep difficulties with health-related quality of life among patients with fibromyalgia. BMC Musculoskelet Disord. 2012;17(13):199.

Weingarten TN, et al. Impact of tobacco use in patients presenting to a multidisciplinary outpatient treatment program for fibromyalgia. Clin J Pain. 2009;25(1):39–43.

Wheatley D. Stress-induced insomnia treated with kava and valerian, singly and in combination. Hum Psychopharmacol. 2001;16:353–56.

Wolfe F, Clauw D, Fitzcharles MA, et al. The American College of Rheumatology preliminary diagnostic criteria for fibromyalgia and measurement of symptom severity. Arthritis Care Res. 2010;62:600–610.

Wolfe F, Hassett A, Walitt B, Michaud K. Mortality in fibromyalgia: A study of 8,186 patients over thirty-five years. Arthritis Care Res. 2011;63(1):94–101.

Wolfe F, Smythe HA, Yunus MB, et al. The American College of Rheumatology 1990 criteria for the classification of fibromyalgia: Report of the Multicenter Criteria Committee. Arthritis Rheum. 1990;33:160–72.

Xiao Y, He W, Russell IJ. Genetic polymorphisms of the beta2-adrenergic receptor relate to guanosine protein-coupled stimulator receptor dysfunction in fibromyalgia syndrome. J Rheumatol. 2011;38(6):1095.

Xiao Y, Russell IJ, Liu YG. A brain-derived neurotrophic factor polymorphism Val66Met identifies fibromyalgia syndrome subgroup with higher body mass index and C-reactive protein. Rheumatol Int. 2012;32(8):2479–85.

Younger J, et al. Low-dose naltrexone for the treatment of fibromyalgia: Findings of a small, randomized, double-blind, placebo-controlled, counterbalanced, crossover trial assessing daily pain levels. Arthritis Rheum. 2013;65(2):529–38.

Zautra AJ, et al. The effects of slow breathing on affective responses to pain stimuli: an experimental study. Pain. 2010;149(1):12–18.

Library and Archives Canada Cataloguing in Publication

McCrindle, Louise S., author
  The complete fibromyalgia health, diet guide & cookbook / Dr. Louise S. McCrindle, B.Sc. (Hons), ND &
Dr. Alison C. Bested, MD, FRCPC.

Includes index.
ISBN 978-0-7788-0453-6 (pbk.)

1. Fibromyalgia—Popular works. 2. Fibromyalgia—Diet therapy.
I. Bested, Alison C., 1953–, author II. Title.

RC927.3.M34 2013   616.7'420654   C2013-903328-9

Index